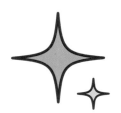

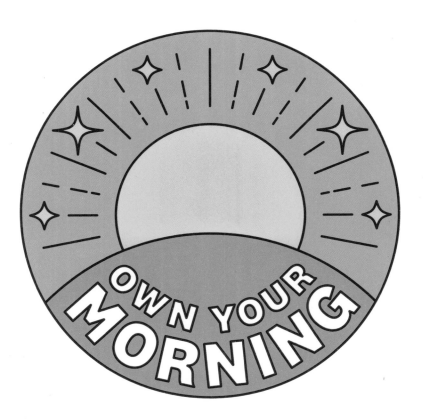
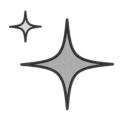

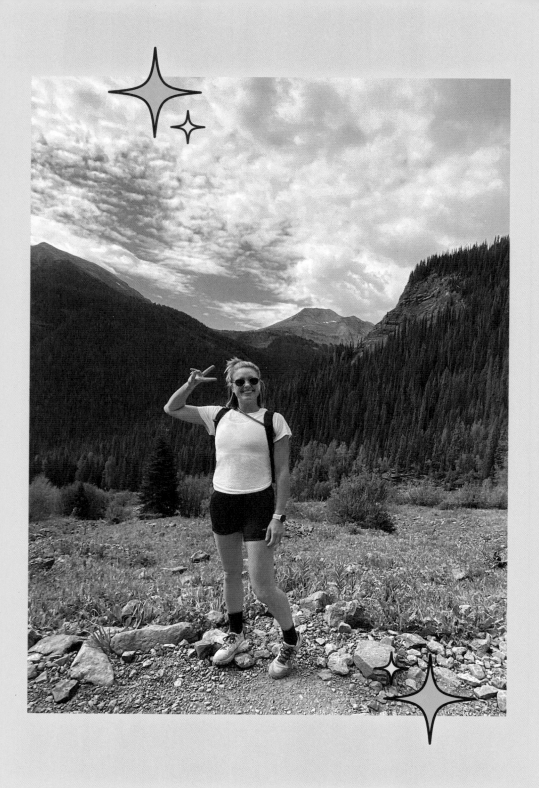

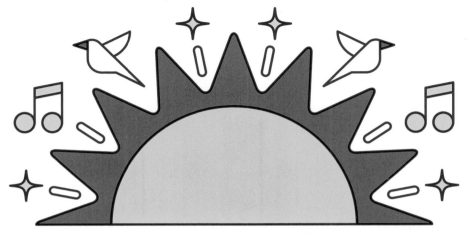

OWN YOUR MORNING

Reset Your A.M. Routine to Unlock Your Potential

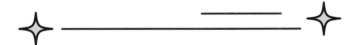

LIZ BAKER PLOSSER

EDITOR-IN-CHIEF OF Women's Health

HEARST
HOME

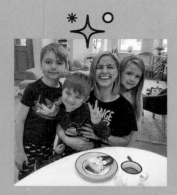
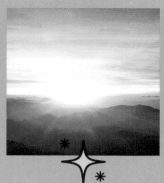
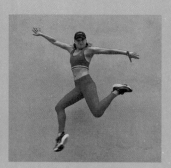
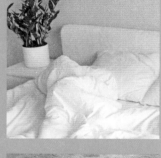

How you start your day? That's how you live your day.

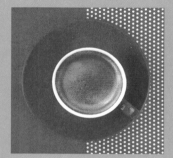
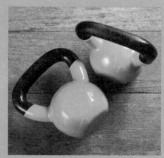
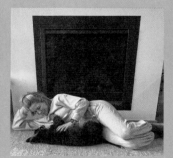
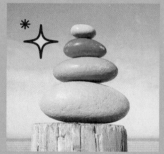
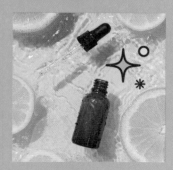
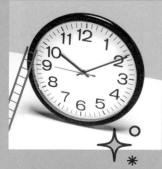
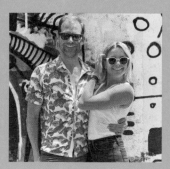

Contents

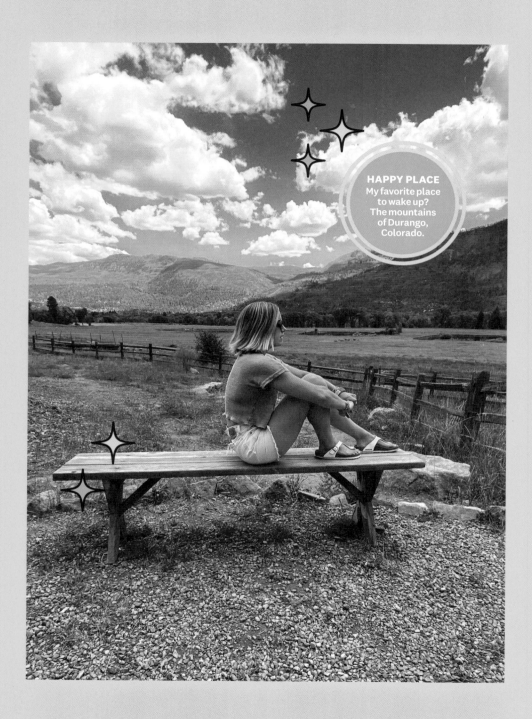

HAPPY PLACE
My favorite place
to wake up?
The mountains
of Durango,
Colorado.

PEOPLE ASK ME ALL THE TIME, "How do you start your day with so much energy and enthusiasm? Where do you find that fire to get after it?" My passion for mornings begins with the knowledge that how I start my day is exactly how I'll live my day. Once you believe that, like I do, you'll do whatever it takes to own your morning.

The truth is, I was *not* born this way. My journey to becoming a morning person reminds me of lifting weights at the gym: The more you flex a muscle, the stronger it becomes. I'm mostly a happy person (phew). But the reality is that I am not a superwoman....I just play one on TV (or more accurately, on my Instagram account!).

Kicking my day off right enables me to give my best effort in each hour that follows. So I am disciplined about my mornings and take care of myself the way I would my three kiddos—boy-girl twins Charlie and Lucy, and their little brother, George.

For example, imagine your child has a soccer game tomorrow morning. Would you let him stay up late watching movies? No way! He'd be rubbing his eyes and weepy from fatigue before the game. Would you walk him out the front door without a healthy breakfast? Absolutely not. He'd have a stomachache from hunger pains. What if you forgo the jacket or sweatpants? Good luck actually making it to soccer if he's cold and uncomfy!

The point is: You'd anticipate everything he needs to feel his best out there...and to minimize the chance of a meltdown along the way. I've learned over time that I am basically a toddler in an adult woman's body. If I'm cold, I'm cranky. If I don't get enough sleep, I'm oversensitive. If I'm hungry, I can't hustle. So I anticipate everything I need to tee up an awesome a.m.

This book is the blueprint to making the most—whatever that means to you—of those first few hours and minutes of your day. In chapters one and two, you'll identify your core values: the ways you spend your energy, time, and resources.

Once you're clear on your values, you'll leverage them to align your morning routine with your goals, hopes, and dreams. The remaining chapters are filled with science-backed suggestions from researchers, doctors, athletes, engineers, actors, poets, and the editors of *Women's Health* for how to do just that. So feel free to read this book choose-your-own-adventure style. Or soak it all up. It's your journey.

But any healthy choice you make is good. So congrats on a very excellent one: reading this book! It means you're already improving your well-being and on the way to owning your morning.

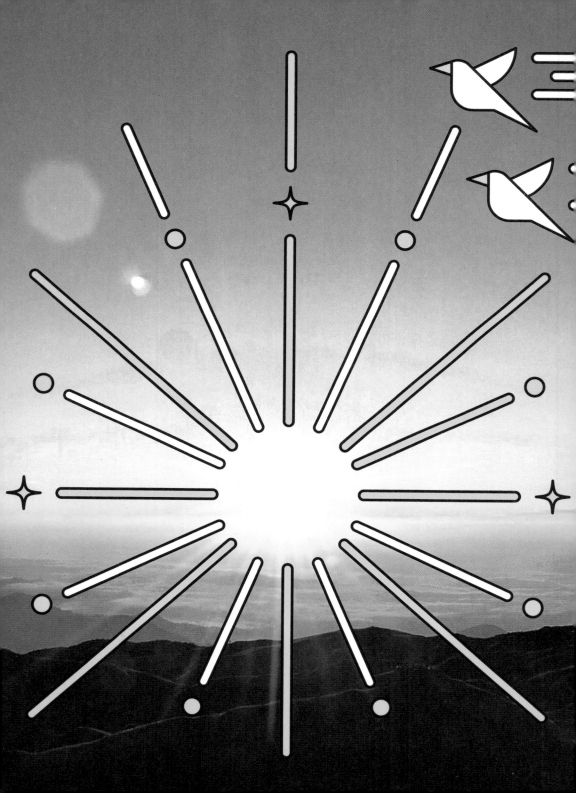

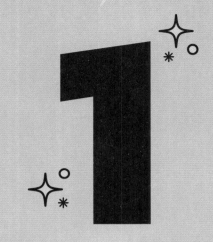

1

You Are a Morning Person

Seriously, anyone can become one.
No matter what your current a.m. routine looks like, you already have the power inside yourself to transform it into a healthier, happier experience. Think of the first few hours after you wake like a warm-up that will prime you for all of the unexpected twists and turns—and possibilities!—that the rest of the day has in store.

The Magic of Mornings

Although I groan at my early alarm just like everyone else (right?!), I'm always better for it when I begin my day before the rest of the city is up.

My ideal morning includes coffee, a bit of work to get a jump start, a feel-good sweat, and some quality (ahem, chaotic) time with my three young children, my husband, and my puppy.

According to my parents, I wasn't always this enthusiastic about mornings. My dad and I still laugh about how the only way he could convince me to jog or play tennis with him before 8 a.m. in high school was if he promised me we'd get a very large latte afterward. (Clearly, coffee has always been nonnegotiable.)

It didn't matter if I promised him the night before that I'd wake up early or if I was training for a big tournament and could use the extra practice. When he came knocking on my door in the morning with a gentle "Lizboo?" it felt impossible to unglue my head from my soft, warm pillow. I know I'm not alone. (Two of my three kiddos are firmly on Team Pillow.) We're not all born morning people, but I'm guessing you wouldn't mind becoming one.

There is hope. Fast-forward to the present, and I am up at 5:17 a.m. most days, ready to get after my to-do list. (Cheerfully, even, once the caffeine kicks in!) Now, I consider owning my morning to be my superpower. And the cool thing is, I can teach you how to do it, too, whether you are starting at ground zero or just want to upgrade your a.m. routine a bit. It's easy to tell yourself you're "not a morning person." And while that may be true (researchers think your DNA might help determine whether you're an early bird or a night owl. Check out "What's Your Chronotype?" on page 13), there are science-backed ways to train yourself to become one.

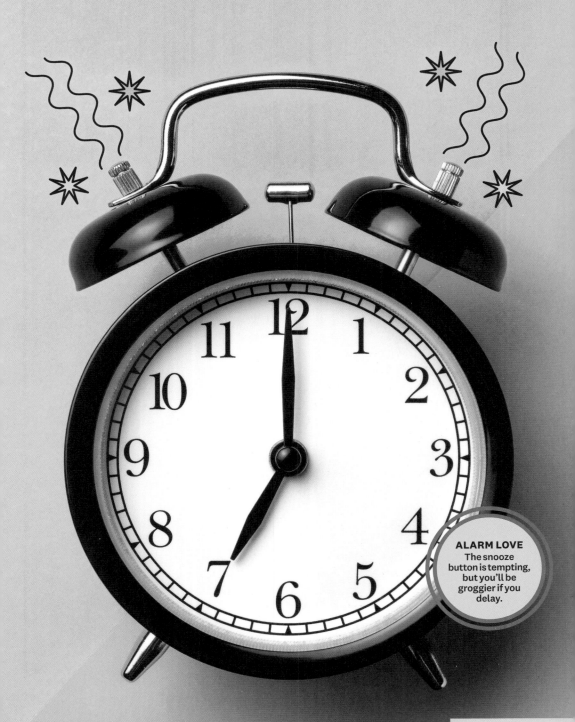

ALARM LOVE
The snooze button is tempting, but you'll be groggier if you delay.

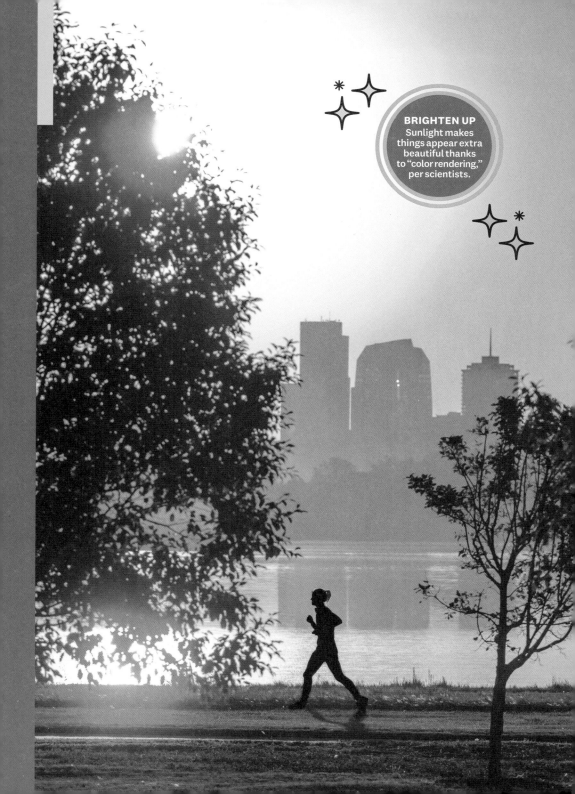

BRIGHTEN UP
Sunlight makes things appear extra beautiful thanks to "color rendering," per scientists.

It doesn't require a super-early alarm, by the way. A friend recently DM'd me a picture of herself in bed, snuggling with her dog, with the hashtag #OwnYourMorning stamped on it. (Hi, Bridget! I love it when followers do this, BTW.) She added the laughing/crying-face emoji, and I did indeed LOL, but the truth is that sometimes sleeping in *is* a version of the perfect morning.

An awesome a.m. doesn't require a workout either. After family pancakes on Saturdays, for example, I might hit a farmers' market, filling a tote bag with deliciousness—fresh produce and herbs. All while sipping an iced coffee with a squirt of chocolate sauce. (I know. Always coffee!) Sometimes a perfect morning involves more sweets than sweat.

The point is, there are all sorts of ways to own your morning, and you are the architect of how it looks and feels. An a.m. victory for you might look like beginning a meditation practice, sipping a mug of tea, walking your dog without being rushed, or getting the kids to school minus any drama.

The first few hours after you wake up are a microcosm of your life, and of the people and things that are important to you. I love how beautifully unique that will look for each of us. This chapter features the varied approaches of powerhouse women—use their stories to spark your own morning magic.

What's Your Chronotype?

Like your wristwatch, your body's master clock ticks away without your being consciously aware of it, directing the release of hormones and chemicals that make you feel sleepy, hungry, alert, and more. When you combine these biochemical signals, your physiological response, and your genetics, you get a chronotype.

Experts tend to use three chronotype categories: **morning types,** or people who naturally wake up early, feel hungry in the morning, and power down relatively easily and early at night; **day types,** who are more likely to enjoy peak alertness a few hours into the day; and **evening types,** who click with Vampire Hours, working and playing into the night.

Many of us switch types throughout our lives, and (*yesss*) going from the day or night category to the morning category is quite common for middle-aged adults. Even better news: You can teach yourself to go to sleep earlier and wake up earlier.

If you're not confident what your chronotype is, try the Center for Environmental Therapeutics' "Your Circadian Rhythm Type" survey at cet-surveys.com.

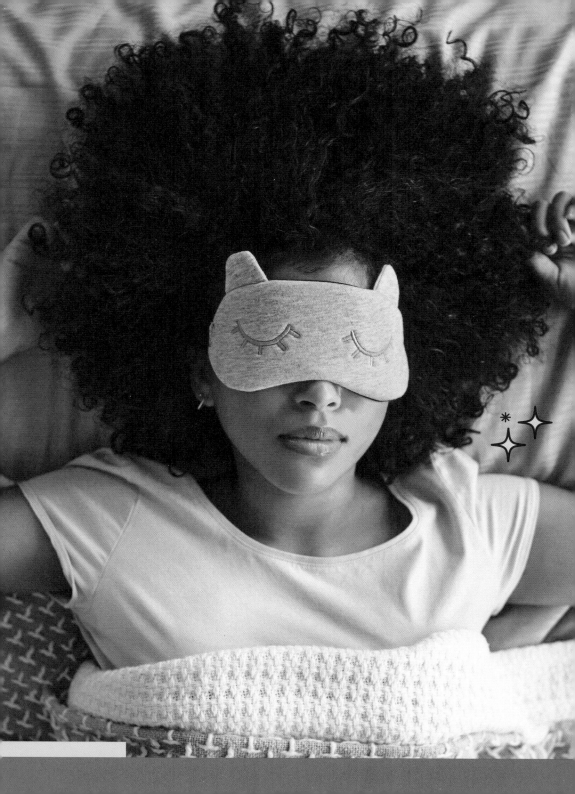

Aspirational Early Birds

●●●

Not a self-described morning person? Even love-to-sleep-in-ers can become dawn patrol members. Take it from these four women, who prove that creating some morning me-time is a game changer.

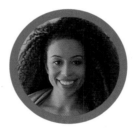

Maud Arnold

Professional tap dancer, producer, and writer

▸ **"I WRITE A HAIKU AS SOON AS I WAKE UP.** I realized I was becoming addicted to waking up and immediately checking my texts, emails, Instagram, and Facebook. Before I had even started my day, my mind was already working on 10 other things for other people. So I wanted to create a low-pressure commitment to myself—something that would activate my brain and make me happy as soon as I woke up. I literally start smiling when I write them. After I write my haiku, I post it on my Instagram Story—I love getting responses from other people sharing their haiku, which has been super unexpected and very cool—and I turn on some music that suits my mood, which ranges from Prince to J. Cole to Michael Jackson to Drake. Then I'm ready to hit a 7 a.m. Cuerpaso workout with my brother, Tadeo."

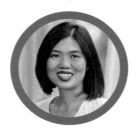

Jeena Cho

Host of the *Resilient Lawyer* podcast and coauthor of *The Anxious Lawyer*

▸ **"I USED TO WAKE UP AND BE IN A FRENZY** to get through everything. I found that hurriedness stuck with me. Now, I'm intentional about self-care with a morning buffer. It helps me recognize that negative thoughts from my inner critic aren't true. I practice insight meditation, which focuses on sensations and thoughts, with the goal of becoming more in tune with reality. I keep it short. When I forget to do it, I don't berate myself. I simply begin again."

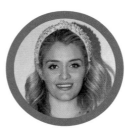

Daphne Oz

Natural-food chef and cookbook author

▸ **"I'M NOT A MORNING PERSON,** but in a perfect world, I'm up at 6 a.m. squeezing in a workout. When I first get up, I try to stream an Our Body Electric class. They're only 28 minutes and you don't need equipment, which means I can do it anywhere I can hide from the children or even when they're climbing all over me. If I can't get a workout in, I'm not too hard on myself. I set the bar low so that if I can do only 10 minutes of stretching, I still feel good about it."

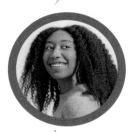

Trinity Mouzon Wofford

Founder of Golde superfood powder tonic and masks

▸ **"AS SOON AS I'M UP,** I pour myself a really big cup of lemon water. I'm usually pretty dehydrated, especially since it gets hot in our tiny apartment. From there, I grab my phone, but I try to limit the screen time to about 15 minutes for emails, social, and the news—otherwise I get sucked in, and the next thing I know, an hour has gone by. If I don't have a lot of time, I'll do 10 to 15 minutes of stretching, but ideally, it's 40 minutes of Yoga With Adriene. Her videos are super approachable and focused on individual exploration as opposed to achieving perfection. Starting my morning by getting in touch with my breath and my body really makes me feel my best and sets a positive tone that helps me tackle whatever's to come. I always take a shower and put on 'work clothes' in the morning to differentiate me-time and business time. It creates a great work persona, and as long as I'm in that, I'm in the zone, even though I'm at home."

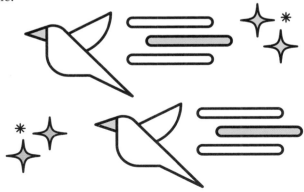

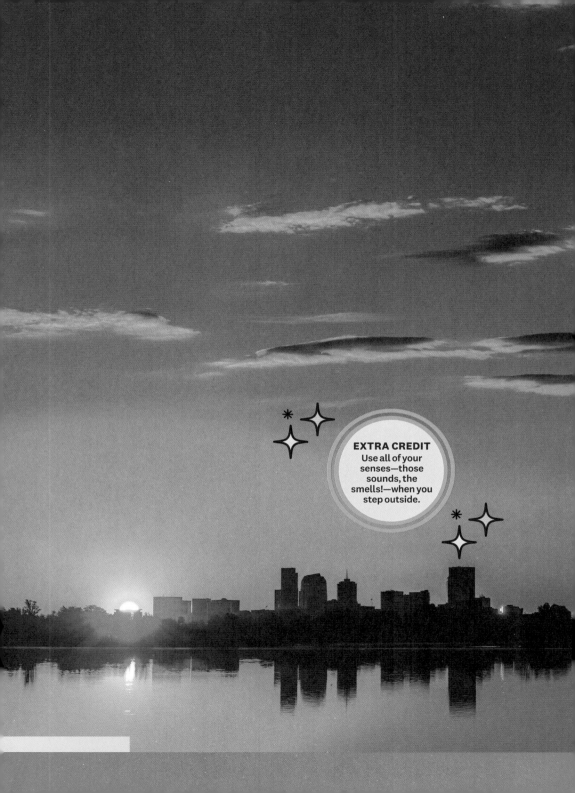

EXTRA CREDIT
Use all of your
senses—those
sounds, the
smells!—when you
step outside.

Rise and Shine

If waking up earlier is important to you, here are research-proven tips to help you make it happen.

1 SET YOUR ALARM WITH SOME INTENTION

Most mornings, I rise with my phone's 5:17 a.m. alarm. Psychologically, the seven gives me a little sense of urgency. If it's 5:00 or 5:15 or even 5:20, I feel like I'd roll over and press snooze because, you know, I've got 5 or 10 more minutes to sleep. (More on snoozing, next column.)

Plus, seven is my lucky number—I was born on April 7—and I love starting my day with its energy. I haven't read a study that confirms this yet, but if there's a certain number that's important to you, I highly recommend giving it some love in the morning.

Pro tip: Choose an alarm sound that makes you happy, rather than the default angry bleep noise. Personally, I love the iPhone's chimes sound. Experiment and find your own fave.

2 DON'T PRESS SNOOZE

Oh, I know. It's so tempting! But the extra few minutes you get between buzzes (or now, hopefully, chimes!) aren't benefiting you much. The "snooze button, pillow, repeat" cycle could even have negative consequences.

"The final stages of your sleep cycle tend to be REM sleep, or dream sleep," says Reena Mehra, MD, the director of sleep disorders research at Cleveland Clinic. "If you're hitting the snooze button, then you're disrupting that important time."

It's not just that your too-early alarm could cause you to lose out on a portion of your most restorative dream state. It's also that disrupting REM sleep can cause a fight-or-flight response in your body, further spiking your blood pressure and heartbeat on top of the blood pressure and heart rate surges naturally occurring during REM sleep. So determine when you absolutely *have to* get up. That, my friends, is your alarm sweet spot.

3 ADD (GOOD!) MOOD LIGHTING

To amp up your alertness first thing, you need to suppress melatonin production in your body. Enter: light! Any kind is helpful, but researchers have determined that certain varieties work best. "A bright, cool, white light is like having a cup of morning espresso," says Hyeon-Jeong Suk, PhD, an associate professor in the department of industrial design at the Korea Advanced Institute of Science and Technology, whose research examines how light affects mood, learning, and more. (This is exactly why you should avoid screens at night, when winding down.) All the better if your bulb includes notes of blue, which has been found to improve mood and focus better than the soft, warm light often found in bedrooms.

Try to get some outdoor light ASAP. "It's a wonderful idea to expose yourself to sunlight first thing," says Dr. Suk. "It's free—and things appear more beautiful under the sunlight." No, seriously: It improves "color rendering," which is a science-y way of saying that stuff looks extra pretty. (Must be why I can't stop taking pictures when I'm out at dawn, and sharing them with a heart-eyes emoji.) More bonuses: An early dose of daylight helps with health issues like insomnia, PMS, and seasonal affective disorder, per studies.

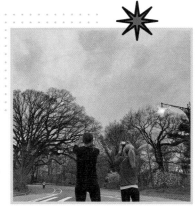

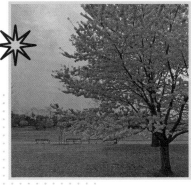

▶ Who can blame me and my friends Kelsy and Brooke for stopping on the run for these pics?

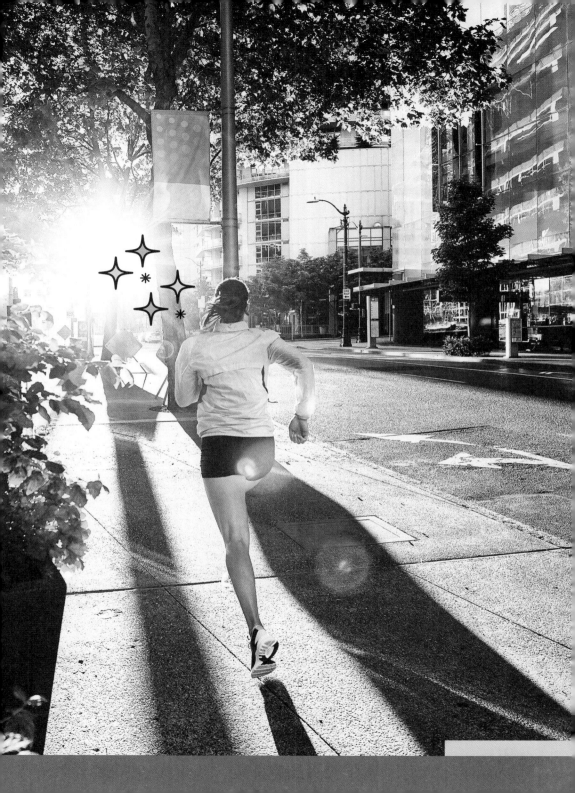

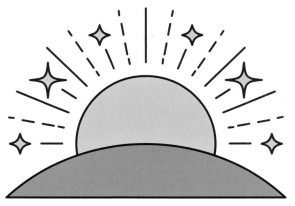

MORNING MAGIC

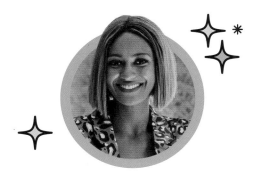

Lauren Maillian, CEO of DigitalUndivided,
the social start-up that leverages data
and advocacy work to create economic pathways
for Black and Latinx women entrepreneurs

KNOW SOME PEOPLE RISE AT 6, 5, OR EVEN 4 A.M., but I own it that some mornings, I'm not up until 8 a.m. I remember when my teenage children were toddlers in nursery school and everyone was desperate for the 9 a.m. spot. Me? I happily took the 1 p.m. afternoon session and enjoyed those unrushed morning cuddles.

It may not be the traditional "type A" morning, but I'm good with that. Great with it, actually. My version of walking? It's everyone else's version of running! Life is so stressful and high-energy that I need my mornings to set the tone for each day: achieving my goals, staying focused, and enjoying what I do.

As soon as I wake up, I want to feel completely supported, as if I'm receiving a hug. Every day is different for me professionally—I might be speaking at a few conferences or leading a large team meeting or attending two networking dinners—so I shape each morning uniquely to power me up for what I need that day.

One constant: I use my five senses (touch, smell, sound, taste, sight) as a form of self-care. My day usually begins with me opening a window to let in fresh air and a gentle breeze. Then it's off to each of my kids' rooms to snuggle with them for 15 minutes. Nope, I haven't let those morning cuddles go.

You know how stores and hotels have signature scents? I created my own for my home: It's lavender- and geranium-based, inspired by our family trips to the South of France, along with some notes of magnolia and hibiscus. It's a sweet, sensual, welcoming smell. Similarly, we have our own "soundtrack" playing in the background: usually soft jazz and soul. The tunes don't require me to think, and they don't distract me. They keep just the right energy.

Meditation is saved for my evenings; my mornings are about energy. I always try to get in an a.m. workout, even if it's just 20 minutes on my Peloton, because moving my body lights me up from the inside out. If I've got an event, I take it up a notch with what I call a "Lights, camera, action!" workout (about 45 minutes longer than my usual 20) to feel extra invigorated.

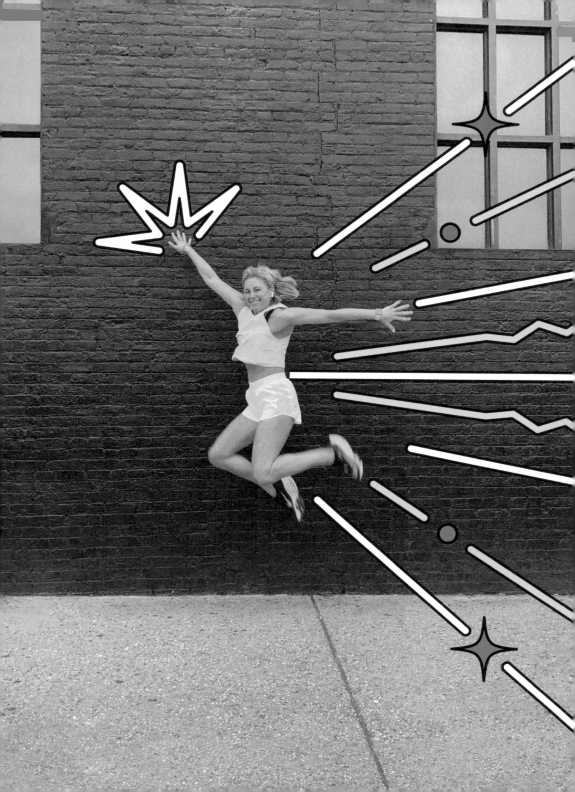

2
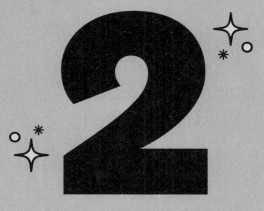

What's Your Perfect Morning?

Everyone's a.m. victory will look a little different.
The goal we all share? To unlock the truest version
of ourselves, starting at sunrise. If you're already in tune
with what sparks your energy, awesome. And if
you're in the dark on that front? I've got you too. This
chapter will help illuminate elements of your
perfect morning that you may not have thought of before.

Learn What Lights You Up

One of my favorite parts of my job is meeting with women—on panels, at events, in interviews for articles—and learning all about their varied morning routines.
I love hearing about the products, apps, food, etc. that folks of all different backgrounds and from a variety of professions turn to as soon as they wake up. It's voyeuristic, and also incredibly inspiring.

Your morning has the potential to express the people, places, things, and feelings that are important to you. But for many of us, the way we spend our time isn't quite aligned with what truly makes our souls happy. This chapter is all about pinpointing where you want to focus your precious energy.

Put another way, you have the opportunity to consciously bring your personal core values to life as your morning unfolds. *Core values* is a term I have been obsessed with since a three-month

leadership training course I took when I worked at SoulCycle, the boutique indoor cycling studio. (FYI: My role was to oversee all the words at the brand, from emails to signage in studio windows. I was most definitely not an instructor. I do love to ride at Soul-Cycle, though!)

The workshop was led by life coach Judy Goldberg, the founder of Wondershift, who works with individuals and businesses to help people perform at their peak and feel their best. My colleagues and I learned a lot about how to give feedback, listen actively, nurture team members, and delegate—all crucial manager skills. Just as important, we learned to identify our personal strengths, weaknesses, and more.

Goldberg's program powerfully impacted me. First of all, she helped me pinpoint my personal core values. Second, she taught me how to do a "wellness check" on them regularly, by asking myself, *Am I living my life in alignment with those values? Have they changed, and do I need to recalibrate accordingly?*

I can tell you that I truly do celebrate my core values, beginning at 5:17 a.m. every morning. You can, too, and it will make you a healthier, happier human. This chapter is about discovering what lights you up so you can intentionally embrace *that* when you roll out of bed.

Time to put pen to paper. (Or fingers to keyboards!) Goldberg and I adapted the following exercises from her coursework to help you identify your own core values. Whether you do all the activities or just one, you'll learn something about yourself that you can immediately apply to your mornings.

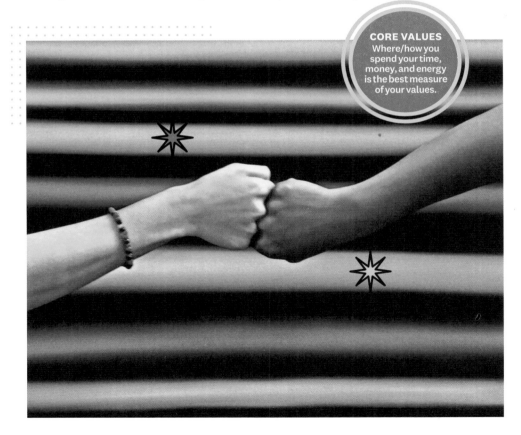

CORE VALUES
Where/how you spend your time, money, and energy is the best measure of your values.

The Calendar Check

▼

For one month, one week, or even just one day, track everything you do in an hour-by-hour calendar or planner. (I used the Microsoft Outlook app.) Eating. Workouts. Helping the kids with homework. Coffee breaks. Laundry. Watching Netflix. The more days you track, the more insight you'll gain into personal behavioral patterns and, subsequently, what's most important to you.

THE TAKEAWAY

Look for themes. Which activities pop up again and again? Circle the repeats. Reflect on them. Those gems are likely the root of your core values. In my calendar, workouts make regular appearances. It's a given that I move my body most days of the week, even if that's just some gentle stretching.

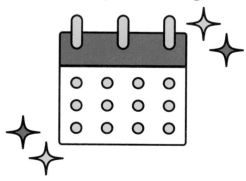

The One-Sheet

▼

Take out a piece of paper and divide it into three columns, with *Time*, *Energy*, and *Money* written at the top. Think about your calendar, your bank account, and your to-do list, and complete a self-inventory in each column as follows....

TIME

Where did you spend your time? How many hours on preparing dinner? How many hours calling family members? How many hours on your exercise bike or streaming yoga?

MONEY

Where did you spend it? Food? Get specific: How much was on groceries? Clothes? Travel? Eating out? The more detailed you are, the easier it is to observe the patterns.

ENERGY

Where do your mental and emotional labor go? This is usually the most difficult column for people to fill in, by the way. You may be thinking, *I spend most of my energy on my job.* Just keep in mind that in, say, an eight-hour workday, you'll spend time doing different things, so try to parse out specific activities where you exert energy. Maybe you

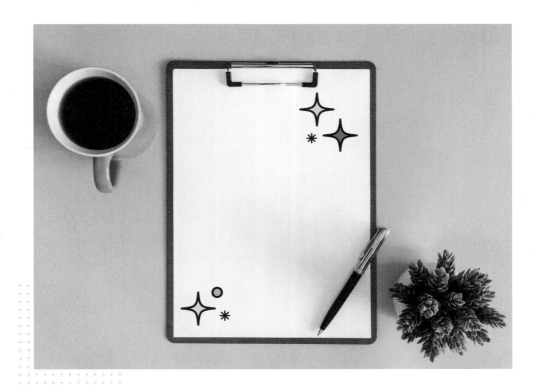

spend half the day on the phone with clients. Maybe you brainstorm—solo or with your team.

THE TAKEAWAY

Explore the items that take up most of each column. When I look at the energy column, I notice I spend the vast majority of my days in meetings with my teammates. The irony is that I consider myself an introvert. So why do I devote so much time to something so...

social? And is my professional life out of sync with my core values?

Nope, says Goldberg. Drill down to analyze the underlying meaning. In my case: I love the vibes that flow when a group of people come together to share ideas. (This is palpable IRL, as well as virtual meetings: I call it Zoomrgy.) When I feel safe to speak freely—and know others do too—it isn't an energy suck. It's invigorating. Ahh, got it. *Collaboration* is a Liz core value!

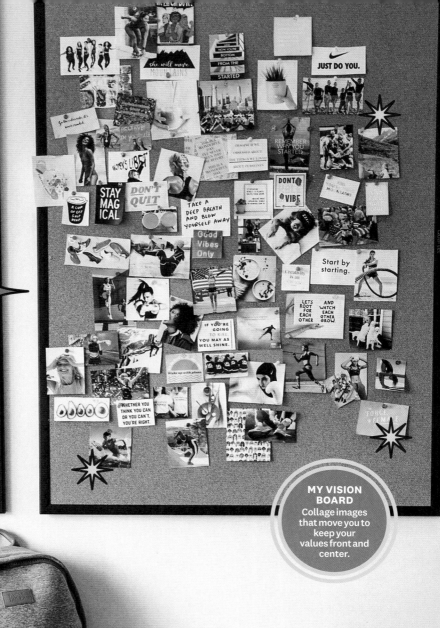

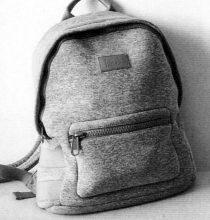

EXERCISE
The Interview

▼

Next, dig in with a trusted friend
or pull out a notebook. You'll
be asking each other (or yourself)
this set of questions.

1. How would you describe your ideal day?
2. What lights you up?
3. What captures your curiosity?
4. What do you love doing so much that
   success or failure doesn't matter?
5. What are you most proud of?
6. What would you drop anything for?

THE TAKEAWAY

Yes, these are deep philosophical
questions. They're also a surefire way to
illuminate passions. Don't be surprised
if whatever captures your curiosity is
something you're not currently explor-
ing. That's normal...and fixable!

As an example, this exercise showed
me that *mentoring* is an unnurtured
core value in my life. It lights me up
to see colleagues soar professionally.
So, I'm newly committed to answering
those cold emails from young women
asking for career advice. It also helped
me realize that I want to give my time
to communities that might benefit from
my experiences. Learning this about
myself inspired me to join the executive
board of the YMCA in New York City.

EXERCISE
Find the Clusters

▼

Review what you wrote and look for patterns. You'll notice certain phrases and
words keep showing up. Maybe your one-
sheet and calendar are filled with words
like *laughter*, *basketball*, *board games*.
(And if so, let's be friends!) Or maybe you
see words like *volunteering*, *marching*,
voting. Take note of those themes.

THE TAKEAWAY

Now, pick a word that describes the
cluster you've identified. And have fun
with it! For the two clusters above, the
words *play* or *impact* might feel right.
And that, my friends, is a core value. So
cool, right?

Now take it a step further and give
your groups of core values a tagline.
Some of mine include *sweat* (which
gives me clarity and focus), *family* (QT
with my husband and children give me
the warm fuzzies), and *teamwork* (collaboration with colleagues, my competitive streak, that mentoring discovery).
So the phrase I use as shorthand for my
core values? "Clear eyes, full heart, can't
lose." Full disclosure: It's a line from the
TV show *Friday Night Lights*, which I
love. Feel free to channel words, colors,
songs, brands, and more that resonate
with you for inspiration.

Align With Your Core Values

▼

This activity is all about identifying the ways you are living and breathing your core values in your life. If *impact* is one of your core values, then reflect on how you brought it to life over the past few months. How many hours did you volunteer? Did you get involved with an org you love? Talk to others about a cause that's important to you? And in that spirit, go ahead and apply this scrutiny to your mornings: Think about how, if at all, you brought a core value to life soon after waking up.

THE TAKEAWAY

Brainstorm ways to ensure your core values show up every morning. If *family* is one of them, I'm not suggesting you find the time to call your sister by 7 a.m. for a marathon catch-up. It can be a micro moment. Kissing a child who's still sleeping in bed, for example, might be a quick but epic nod to it.

Maybe *food* or *wellness* is one of your core values. Simply having a bowl of fresh green apples on your kitchen counter that you see as soon as you're up and at 'em integrates that passion into your morning. If, like me, *sweat* is what gets you going, hopefully you can find a way to work out most mornings.

The point is, it can be tiny (a kiss on the cheek, the bowl of apples) or T. rex (like a five-mile run). It all counts.

Now that you know your core values, I'm going to let you in on a little secret. They will evolve! So it's ideal to continue revisiting them, especially whenever you're navigating a life transition, like a new job, a move, starting a family, or any other threshold moment. And when something major happens in the world—no shortage of that lately—it's another good time to check in.

Finally, whenever you're feeling stuck in a rut, consider it a signal that it's time to take a look under the hood and see if your core values have shifted. "For people who are drifting or bored or lost, I say, 'Let's do a values exercise!'" says Goldberg. "We tend to make decisions based on perceptions rather than our own internal compass, and 'tuning' your compass will direct you toward a life with purpose and direction."

Another common question: "How many core values should I have?" There's no perfect number, but Goldberg recommends targeting three to seven so you can truly focus on each and every one. Remember that there's no right or wrong core value. They are not meant to be judged by others (or by you!). Embrace yours. And leverage them to help you define your perfect morning.

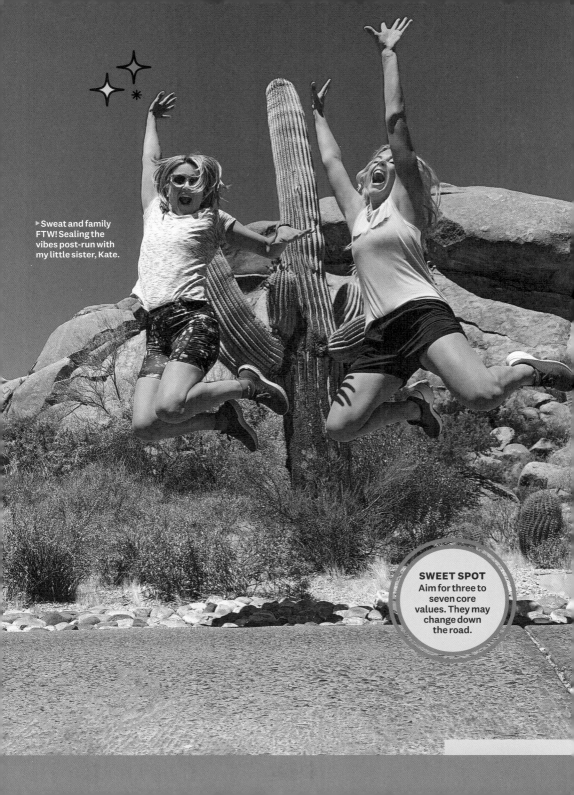

▶ Sweat and family FTW! Sealing the vibes post-run with my little sister, Kate.

SWEET SPOT
Aim for three to seven core values. They may change down the road.

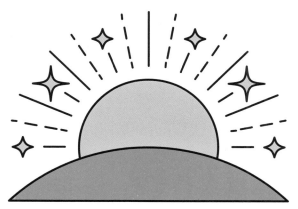

MORNING MAGIC

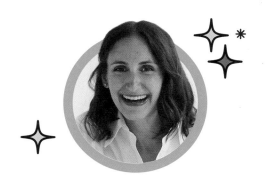

Sofia Adler,
astrologer and life coach

IF I'M BEING HONEST, I've never really felt like I fit in. I wish I could say that I've always been unfazed by what other people think or what society suggests is "cool" in the moment...but that just wouldn't be true.

Instead, I spent years morphing into a version of myself that I didn't like but thought would make me more accepted, appealing, and valuable to others. I said yes to happy hours (even though I prefer intimate settings over big groups). I ordered a glass of wine on first dates (even though I don't like to drink). I stayed in my stable, coveted position at an idolized brand (even though I knew in my gut that a corporate setting was wrong for me).

I was so focused on being who I *thought* I was supposed to be that I lost sight of who I was.

But then life threw me a major curveball. After returning home from a trip to Europe, my parents broke the news: "We're getting a divorce." Feeling gutted, untethered, and incredibly alone, my focus shifted basically overnight from caring about everyone else to keeping myself afloat. I made many changes during that time that impacted the woman I am today.

The biggest, most impactful shift? Reclaiming my love for the mornings. Each morning at dawn—blinds all the way up, eyes on the horizon, hot water with lemon in hand—I reveled in the quiet and turned my focus inward. I allowed myself to move slowly. To meditate. To ponder. To uncover what I really want and what I hoped would happen next—in life, at work, in relationships, and more. I allowed myself permission to drop the "shoulds."

Mornings helped me discover—and empowered me to be, completely and wholeheartedly and unabashedly— myself. Day after day, I used this time to realign with my inner compass and ensure that my values and dreams drove my decisions.

It's how I mustered up the courage to leave my cushy job and go back to graduate school. To leap into the unknown and start my own business. To sit with, own, and honor my discomfort in said business when I knew it wasn't an authentic expression of who I am. To follow my heart yet again, pivot, and incorporate astrology into my work. (Where I learned, by the way, that I have a ton of Aquarius in my chart—i.e., I'm not meant to fit in!)

There's so much in life we can't predict or know for sure. But I'm confident in this: As long as I have the early mornings, whatever path I take will be true to who I am, to what matters to me, and to the kind of life I want to lead.

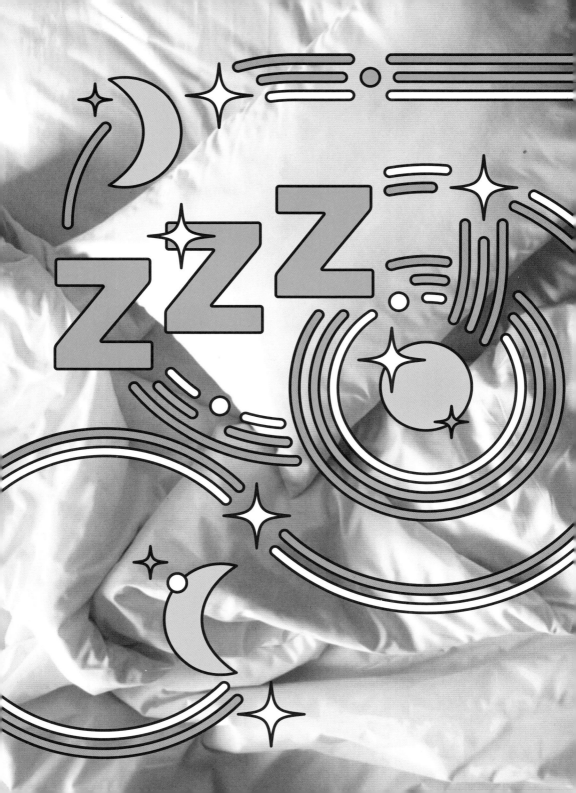

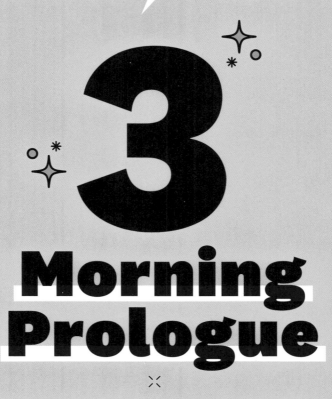

3

Morning Prologue

Let's talk about your evening routine.
And yes, I know how strange it must sound to devote
an entire chapter in a book about mornings to
nighttime. But the truth is that an amazing a.m. begins
many hours before your alarm clock rings. It's not
just about banking a solid, restorative night of sleep. It's
about looking out for your future self—your tomorrow
self—with some simple routines the night before. Putting
each of your a.m. ducks in a row is the most crucial
piece to feeling and being your best. Time to break it down.

Pick Tomorrow's Outfit Tonight

I fully endorse anything that makes it easier to streamline your morning, including picking your outfit the night before. For those of you who work out in the a.m., the same goes for your fitness clothes.

It takes us an average of 17 minutes to pick our clothing in the morning, according to a recent survey. Add that up over the course of the year and we're talking four days' worth of time spent on outfit selection.

You don't lose just precious time from your a.m. by spending it looking through your drawers, by the way. You use up brainpower with every decision you make, according to scientists at the American Psychological Association. Your brain gobbles up glucose (energy!) every time you make a choice. This is probably one reason why Steve Jobs, the cofounder of Apple, had that famous go-to look: black turtleneck, jeans, sneakers.

Personally, my style is more sporty—I love to play with stripes, pops of color, and sneakers, for instance—but I'd rather fatigue my neurons on the stuff that could really benefit from my undivided attention, rather than on outfit selection.

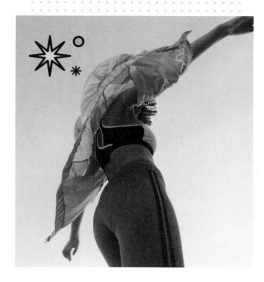

Look Out For Your Future Self

All right, you've got your fitness clothes—sneakers included—ready to rock. Whatever you're planning to wear for work is hanging or neatly folded. You're 90 percent of the way there.

If you're looking for extra credit—and of course you are!—then take it a step further and straighten up your kitchen and countertops before hitting the sack. Believe me, the last thing I want to do is tackle a sink brimming with dirty dishes after getting home from work, making dinner, and tucking the kids into bed. But actually, there is something that sounds even more dreadful: waking up to that mess! Gah, the worst.

On nights I'm really dragging, I imagine my future self—me, tomorrow morning—arriving at an empty, sparkling sink with my mug of coffee in my hand. (Because obviously, I was looking out for Future Liz and set up my coffee maker the night before.)

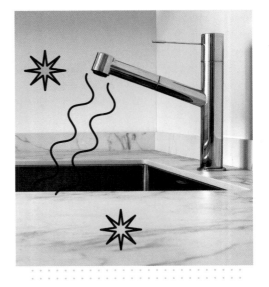

Now that the kitchen is clean, tomorrow's clothes are good to go, and the coffee is ready, you have earned an awesome night of sleep. Everything you need to know to set up for a restorative rest comes next.

The Wind-Down

•••

Taryn Toomey, the founder of The Class, works *hard*. As the creator of a global fitness modality that blends high-intensity training with mindfulness, she teaches multiple classes a week (often as the sun is rising), oversees a team of instructors dispersed across the country, and constantly evolves her brand's streaming and IRL platforms. She puts every cell of her being into it all, which helps hundreds of thousands of people live healthier, happier lives. Scratch that—she also spends tons of energy raising her two young daughters.

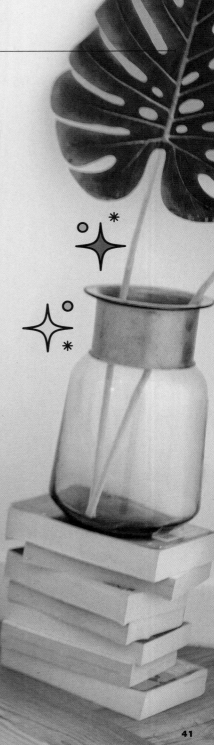

▸ **IT'S ALL INCREDIBLY INVIGORATING BUT ALSO...EXHAUSTING.** "I've started a consistent evening ritual to set myself up to rest well," says Toomey. "We all hear about how important sleep is, and once you know, *you know*." The rituals below help her snooze more soundly while honoring "what sleep does for one's overall mental, emotional, and physical well-being."

1 ONE HOUR PRIOR TO GETTING IN BED, I take a magnesium supplement that helps relax my body.

2 I CHECK EMAILS, texts, and apps before getting into the shower or bath. It's my final moment for all gadgets and devices. I turn off my phone and put it away so I can really slow down and close off feedback from the outside world.

3 I DO SOME SORT OF WATER RITUAL to reset physically, emotionally, and mentally. Taking a bath or shower is a literal and figurative way to "rinse off" my day. I find this incredibly important because I believe we collect our day on our bodies, and it's crucial to create a clean slate.

4 I CRAWL INTO BED AND READ FOR A BIT. When my mind settles, I spin around and put my legs up vertically on my headboard for 10 minutes. I place my hands on my body and allow them to follow my breath. I use this time to take stock of my day, not obsessing or analyzing...simply noticing. It's my moment of reflection. From there, I lie down and rest.

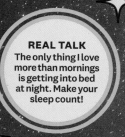

REAL TALK
The only thing I love
more than mornings
is getting into bed
at night. Make your
sleep count!

Secrets to Sleeping Soundly

•••

Claudia Aguirre, PhD, is a neuroscientist and mind-body expert who advises global corporations on wellness. She is also on the *Women's Health* advisory board and chatted with me on the science of sleep.

WHY IS SLEEP SO, SO IMPORTANT?

▸ It's the only way your brain can clear its daily waste. Every single time you think, breathe, work, or even just sit there spacing out, your brain is hard at work. This work leads to a sort of pollution. Think of it like a car: When it's turned on, fumes come out of the exhaust pipe.

Now imagine this car is on, parked inside a closed garage. That is your brain at night. You need to open the windows and let out the polluted air and clean it up. Sleep is like that open window: It allows for the cleaning, decluttering, and refreshing of the brain.

IS IT FAIR TO SAY THAT SLEEP HELPS KEEP US STRONG AND HEALTHY?

▸ Yes. We used to think the blood-brain barrier (BBB) prevented the brain from being "infected" by bodily microbes. In a sense, the BBB protects the brain and keeps nasties at bay. But some things do cross the barrier, like alcohol, and the barrier is not so much a wall as a membrane. Losing sleep could make this membrane weak, which can allow microbes to penetrate the brain if there is a bodily infection.

ANY TIPS FOR READJUSTING SLEEP SCHEDULES SO WE'RE NOT ZOMBIES WHEN THE MORNING ALARM GOES OFF?

▸ Treat your ideal wake-up time like you are flying to a far-off destination. To avoid jet lag, you want to adjust your sleep schedule a bit each night so you wake up closer to the time you're aiming for. Take it night by night so getting out of bed won't be such a struggle.

For me personally, it helps to plan a little something to look forward to in the morning. Maybe it's the promise of a solo meditation session or the new fitness class you're streaming.

ARE THERE ANY SCIENCE-BACKED TIPS FOR SLEEPING BETTER?

▸ First of all, avoid blue light from electronics as much as possible in the evening because it is basically morning light. (See "Blue Light 101" at right.) This helps your brain produce the right hormones that slow your racing mind naturally and help you fall asleep.

Develop a soothing sleep ritual: For example, light a candle to get your brain into the relaxation zone. Then do some breathwork—such as inhaling for four counts, holding for four counts, and then exhaling for four counts, for instance—which helps to flush the cerebrospinal fluid and improve oxygenation. (More on breathwork on page 96.)

I also recommend focusing on a sensory channel, like your skin. A warm bath before bed raises your body temperature enough so that an hour or two after the bath or shower, your core temperature dips, promoting better sleep. Add some magnesium salts and you could be on your way to a deeper sleep. See "The Wind-Down" on page 40 for a inspiring evening bedtime ritual.

IS IT OKAY THAT I LOVE A COLD ROOM?

▸ That's good! We should keep our bedrooms at 68 degrees or less. You can also try a thinner quilt and breathable bedsheets in a cooling fabric like lyocell (a form of rayon) instead of cotton or flannel.

I CAN'T. FALL. ASLEEP. HELP!

▸ Give yourself a good 15 minutes to try to fall asleep. If that doesn't work, get up: Try not to spend too much time in bed awake. This could create a mental signal that your bed isn't for sleeping.

DO YOU SUGGEST SLEEP-PROMOTING FOODS, DRINKS, OR SUPPLEMENTS?

▸ Functional foods like milk, nuts, tart cherry juice, and kiwifruit have been shown to promote healthier sleep. Also: serotonin (5HTP), melatonin, and magnesium can help. Ask a doctor what's right for you.

Blue Light 101

How much time do you spend on your iPad, laptop, and phone as you're winding down for bed? A ton of research suggests this could be damaging to the quality of your sleep. And nope, not just for the obvious reason—that scary stuff spikes your heart rate, making it harder to relax and ultimately preventing you from banking solid shut-eye. It's also because the blue light emanating from your electronic screen has been shown to slow the release of the sleep hormone melatonin. It alters the body's circadian rhythm, which is our wake-and-sleep cycle. During the day, blue light is supposed to wake us up, but exposure at night can make us have some difficulty getting to sleep. Pop on some blue-light-blocking glasses, which boosted sleep quality for participants in a study from the University of Houston. Or shut down your devices at least an hour before bed.

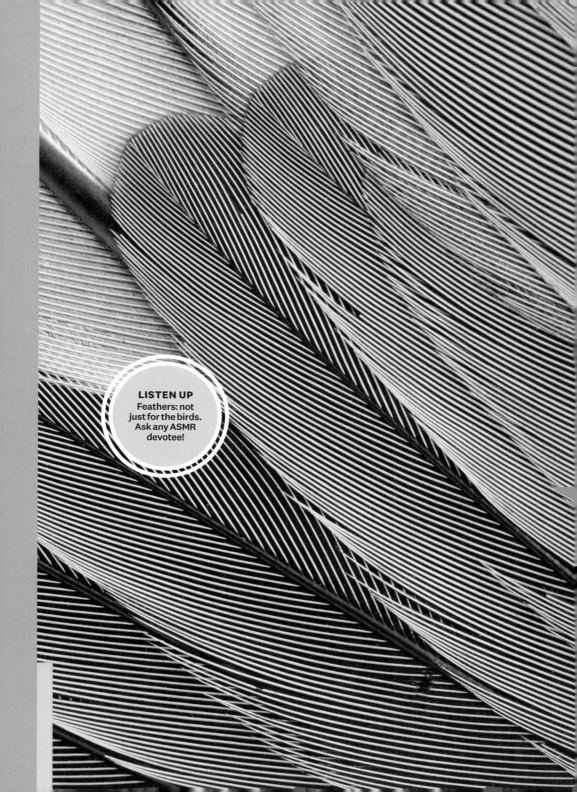

LISTEN UP
Feathers: not
just for the birds.
Ask any ASMR
devotee!

An Alternative Way to Find *Ahh*?

•••

One very nontraditional health fix you def won't find on any treatment list: **ASMR.** In fact, the main place you will find it is on YouTube. Millions of people are turning to it for help with sleep and stress issues, among other problems. The abbreviation stands for "autonomous sensory meridian response," and the videos involve people speaking softly or even moving a makeup brush across a microphone.

▸ **WHY ARE SO MANY FOLKS INTO IT?** ASMR is a sensation triggered by gentle sounds (whispering, crinkling, tapping), light touches, or fluid movements that create a dreamy experience that can feel like tingles all over your body, says ASMR researcher Craig Richard, PhD, a professor of biopharmaceutical sciences at Shenandoah University. Think of it as a digital, drug-free version of chill-out pills. If you think it sounds wacky...but also a little bit lovely? You're not alone. (See "Morning Magic," page 49, for a first-person take on how relaxing it can be.) "It's blissful—and it's totally bizarre because you can get this very real response just by watching videos," Richard says. If you want to see if it has any effect on you, log on to YouTube, check out a few different ASMRtists, and see what happens. "ASMR videos are kind of like a big buffet," Richard says, meaning you may have to sample a bunch of clips with different types of triggers and sounds to see what relaxes you. He recommends the channels Gentle Whispering ASMR, Tony Bomboni ASMR, and Deep Ocean of Sounds.

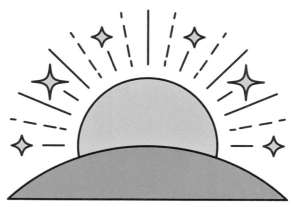

MORNING MAGIC

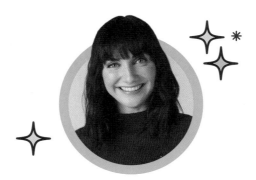

Kristin Canning,
senior editor, *Women's Health*

INSOMNIA RUNS IN MY FAMILY. We're all naturally night owls. But I know how important it is to get to sleep at a decent time if I want to have a happy and productive morning. In my quest to make falling asleep easier and to drown out the city sounds on the other side of my apartment window, I started listening to music and calming nature-sounds videos in bed.

These videos were too jarring to sleep to, but they led me to ASMR videos on YouTube (for more on ASMR, turn to page 47). Performed by ASMRtists, ASMR videos can trigger calming sensations with their soothing sounds and visuals, which help the millions of people who watch and listen chill out and fall asleep faster.

The first time I listened to a video from Gentle Whispering ASMR (a favorite of mine!), I felt a warm wave of relaxation roll over my body. It was euphoric—I felt as if I'd stumbled upon some type of serenity-inducing drug, but I was just listening to a woman talking softly about nothing in particular, scratching her nails on a crinkly pillow, and tapping on a comb inside a plastic wrapper.

Look, I know it sounds weird. It is weird! But these videos force me to tune in to one sense and focus on the subtle changes in timbre between sounds, and that mindfulness gets me out of anxious thought spirals and puts me in a better headspace for sleep. I swear I can feel my blood pressure lowering when I hear one of my go-to voices; it's like a familiar friend, who happens to have the most zen energy, tucking me into bed at night.

Now, I have several ASMRtists in my rotation for different moods—some create unique sounds that feel sort of like a brain massage; others offer feel-good affirmations and comfort. I look forward to their new videos so much that I'm excited to get to bed and drift off, something I never looked forward to before. I've been using ASMR for three years now, and I no longer stress about being able to catch some Zs when I want to. Knowing I have my nighttime self-care ritual (and actual rest!) coming my way makes it so much easier to get up the next morning.

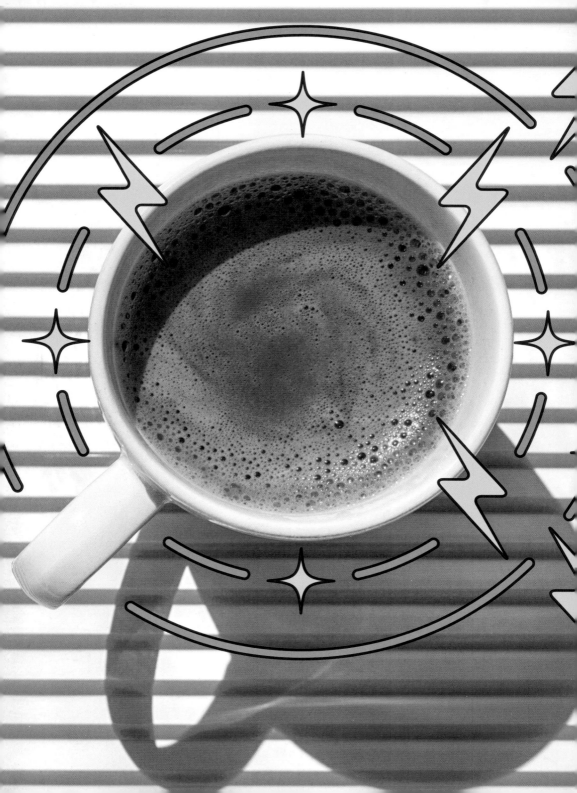

4

Power Breakfasts

Fuel your a.m. awesomeness.

A moment of respect for the first few sips and bites that go into your mouth each day: They're the keys to performing at your peak. But this chapter is about more than just your health, nutrition, and energy levels. Food should also be delicious and make you oh-so-happy. As a recovering sugary-cereal devotee (another story for another time), I promise you can have the best of all of these worlds.

Ace Your A.M.

There is one nonnegotiable to my mornings: coffee. I love each step of the process: hearing it brew in my coffee maker, pouring the piping-hot liquid from the carafe into my mug, warming my hands around it, inhaling the aroma, then taking that first sip. And especially the part when, like magic, my mental fog dissipates. Sigh of contentment; repeat.

I've been a coffee drinker since high school, and I trace it back to morning runs with my dad. In my teenage years, he would convince me to get out of bed and join him for a few miles of jogging by promising me a latte at local Kansas City coffee shops, which doubled as that a.m.'s finish line.

Nowadays, I would never attempt to work out in the morning—or do anything else, actually—without first prepping a hot, caffeinated beverage to get me going. I switched to decaf while I was pregnant with my kiddos—a time when doctors suggest limiting your caffeine intake—and learned that it's as much about the ritual of morning coffee—the brewing, the aroma, the smell—as it is about coffee itself. I discovered that in desperate times, I can swap in decaf or tea and still experience that satisfying sense of my clarity sharpening with each sip.

I know lots of people who opt for hot water with a squeeze of fresh lemon to gently awaken their brains and bodies. Others love smoothies to fuel up for the day. Some dig into a wholesome bowl of overnight oats. Whatever makes you excited to get out of bed is how you should start your day. Embrace the anticipation of those morning sips or bites.

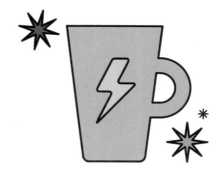

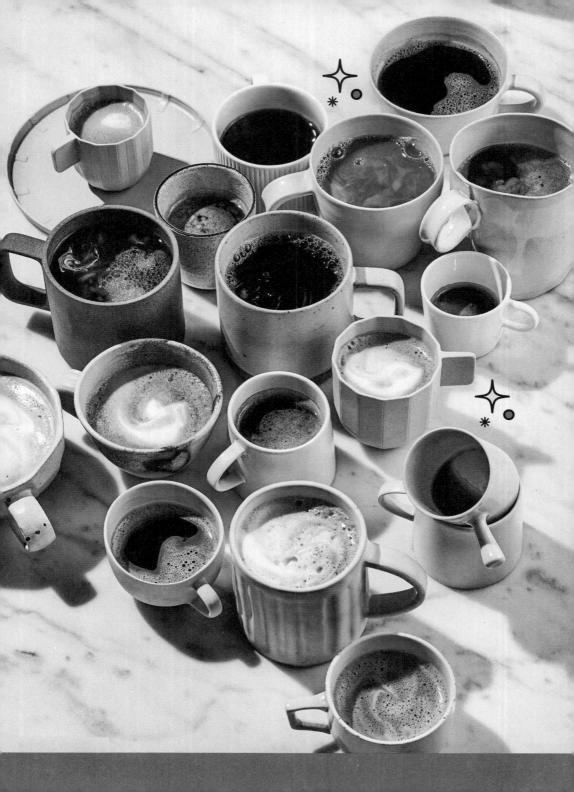

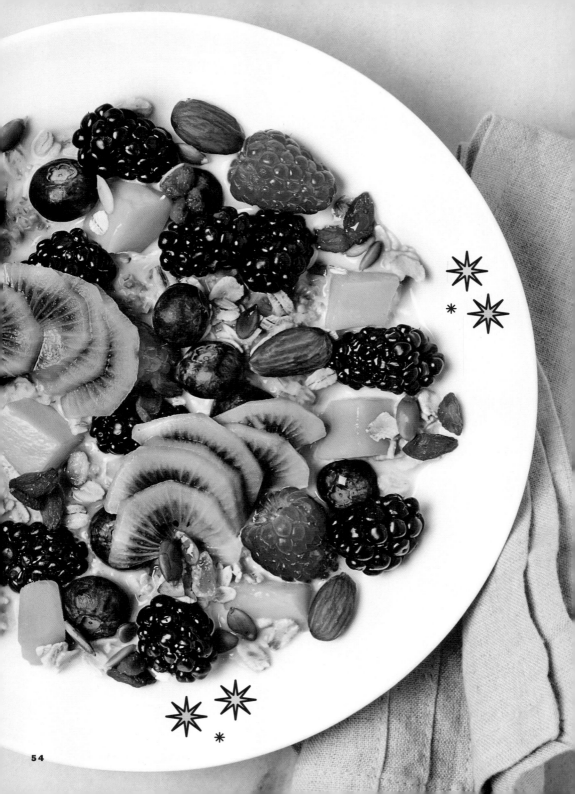

To Breakfast or Not to Breakfast

There's a solid chance you know someone who swears by intermittent fasting. Also known as IF, intermittent fasting describes the method of skipping food and drink (except for water, coffee, and tea) for an extended period of time (think eight hours or more). Research shows that fasting may reduce belly fat, lower your risk for diabetes, and improve brain function. Some superfans of IF even report experiencing glowier skin.

"The goal is to give your body additional time to break down and go through carbohydrate stores so it can turn to burning fat," says Robin Berzin, MD, the founder of Parsley Health and a *Women's Health* advisory board member. "When we fast, insulin—a hormone that allows cells to take in glucose—decreases, which facilitates fat burning. Lowering insulin causes cells to release stored glucose as energy, and repeating this leads to weight loss."

Still, research doesn't suggest that this method is any better for weight loss than other diets. In fact, IF had weight-loss results similar to a traditional calorie-restricted plan in a recent study. Plus, "some people may experience weight loss in the short term, but many people gain that weight back eventually," says NYC-based dietitian Alissa Rumsey, RD, owner of Alissa Rumsey Nutrition and Wellness and author of *Unapologetic Eating*.

And it's definitely not for everyone. Fasting can affect blood sugar and hormone levels, so skip if you have low blood sugar, diabetes, thyroid issues, or gallbladder disease. It could also trigger an underlying eating disorder, so avoid if you have a history of one. Pregnant women and those who are breastfeeding or trying to get pregnant should also skip this trend.

I'll leave you with a strong PSA: Focus on fueling yourself so you can perform at your best! The truth is that there's no magic-bullet trend. It's all about figuring out what works for you, and everyone is different.

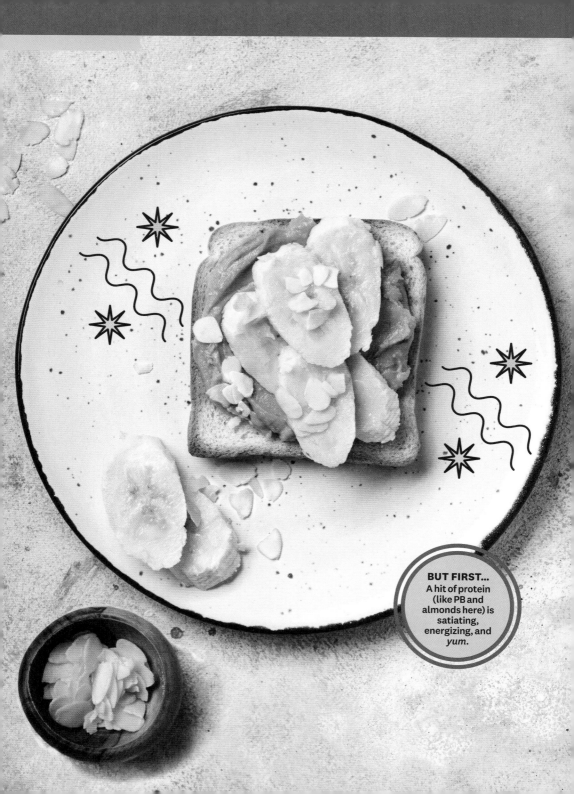

BUT FIRST...
A hit of protein (like PB and almonds here) is satiating, energizing, and *yum*.

Real Talk on Eating and Exercise

•••

Cara Clark, RD, coauthor of *The Wellness Remodel* shares the science behind when and how much to eat if you sweat in the morning. P.S. Clark is also a former collegiate basketball star...such a *WH* girl.

DO I NEED TO EAT BEFORE MY MORNING WORKOUT?

▸ Nope, it's a personal preference. Consider these factors: how hungry you feel, your individual needs, the type of exercise you're going to do, and, most important, your ability to digest food.

Clark's advice: Take into account how long you're going to sweat. If your morning workout is intense (e.g., HIIT or an indoor cycling session) or lasts longer than 45 minutes, she says to grab a snack.

WHAT ABOUT THE CONCEPT OF "FASTED CARDIO"?

▸ This is a term for doing an aerobic workout without eating anything beforehand. "Exercising in a fasted state is often called the 'fat-burning zone' because the body turns to fat for fuel when glucose is not sufficient," says Clark. "Your body's supply of glucose is severely depleted after a night of sleep, so morning exercisers can quickly get into this state." But if you feel weak without a pre-snack? Have one!

WHAT SHOULD I EAT IF I DO NEED A LITTLE SOMETHING TO GET MOVING?

▸ Choose simple carbohydrates that break down quickly and easily, plus small amounts of protein and fat. (If you have a meal with lots of protein and fat—nutrients that take longer to digest—it can lead to bloating and cramping.) Some suggestions from Clark: almonds and a small orange; toast (or a banana) plus peanut butter; applesauce and fruit strips (also called fruit leathers). Carbs are the ideal macronutrient for powering through a workout and keeping your energy up while you sprint or crank out strength reps, then your muscles will use protein afterward to repair, according to Clark.

DO I NEED TO WAIT AFTER EATING TO START MY WORKOUT?

▸ That depends on how well you take in food, says Clark. And everyone is different! If you feel okay to start exercising right after you eat, go for it. But if your stomach tends to feel off mid-sweat—rumbly, crampy, side stitches—try waiting at least 30 minutes.

"Pay close attention to what goes on and how your body reacts during the workout," Clark says. Ask yourself: *Do I have more energy? Can I push harder? Any discomfort? Bathroom breaks?* Experiment to learn what works best for your body.

COFFEE BEFORE SWEAT: YEA OR NAY?

▸ It's a big yes in my book. Coffee before a morning workout intensifies the fat-burning that happens during your workout. Plus, it adds some extra adrenaline. Just be cautious about, er, digestive issues—test it out with a home workout first.

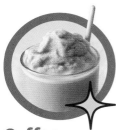

Coffee Smoothie

×

Katrina Scott, the cofounder of Tone It Up—a wellness-focused community of more than a million women—is a self-proclaimed breakfast superfan. Here's her go-to smoothie recipe featuring, yep, coffee.

Serves: 1
Total: 5 min

▸ In a blender, add 1 shot **espresso**, 1 cup **milk of choice** (Scott prefers almond), 1 frozen **banana,** 1 scoop **protein powder** (Scott recs Tone It Up Perfect Protein), and a handful of **unsweetened coconut shavings.** Blend until smooth, and serve.

A Word on Alcohol

×

"I'm never drinking again." Ever uttered that sentence? You, me, and everyone. The love-hate relationship with alcohol is real—and it's why more and more folks are joining the sober-curious movement, or proactively drinking less as they experience the benefits of stepping back from drinking culture (increased energy, less hangover anxiety, better workouts).

Once I dipped my toe into booze-free waters, I felt so good that it might as well have been a cannonball-level jump. When I stopped sipping wine, margs, and other alcoholic drinks, I woke up feeling extra awesome. I gained clarity and calm, discovered that I could be more focused and engaged with my kiddos, my husband, my friends, my work...and I channeled a new level of confidence. (The clincher: I rocked a major presentation a couple of months into my teetotaling and never looked back.) Cheers to all that!

The number of people dabbling in booze-free sips is growing. Mocktail variations on offer at the top 500 full-service chains in the U.S. increased 13 percent in the first half of 2018 compared with the same period in 2016, according to Technomic, a research and consulting firm. And industry trend tracker IWSR Drinks Market Analysis forecasts that consumption of low- and no-alcohol products in the U.S. will grow by 35 percent by 2023.

Informal programs like Sober October and Dry January—where folks nix alcohol for a month—are also helping the trend catch on, says Rachel E.K. Freedman, PhD, a psychologist in Bethesda, Maryland. "For some people, the idea of quitting permanently is really overwhelming or they have ideas tied up with what it means to be sober: 'How will I ever have fun again?' or 'What will people think?'" says Freedman. "But quitting for one month is seen as doable."

▸ **MY ADVICE** If you're curious, just give it a go. You're always allowed to change your mind...and you'll gain some perspective about what you do and don't like about alcohol along the way.

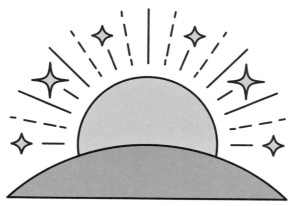

MORNING MAGIC

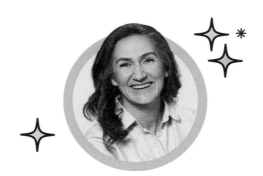

Kate Merker,
chief food director, *Women's Health*

MY BODY WAKES NATURALLY between 5:30 and 6 a.m., which comes in handy with two young kids. But it's really the breakfast routine that I look forward to most....

Which brings me to toast. You might not think toast sounds like the most exciting meal, but bear with me here. It's a metaphor for morning eats: You can take the most standard meal and turn it into an experience, a ritual that will restore, refresh, and help you set up your day for success.

I've always made some version of toast and gradually elevated it along the way. (Note: This was before avo toast was a thing.) The right bread, dark and crusty, cut about three-quarters of an inch to an inch thick, toasted so the outside is crisp but the inside still has some chew to it. Sautéed greens (could be chard, dandelion, spinach, really anything), until they're beginning to wilt. Roasted mushrooms and an egg, fried so the edges are brown and crackly and the white is set but the yolk is bright, beautiful, and jiggly. On the side, a tomato salad with scallions, simply tossed with olive oil, salt, and pepper. That's my idea of perfection. Just thinking about all this makes my mouth water.

I love the beautiful rhythm amidst the chaos in the a.m. of my family gathering around the dining table. We come together around one not-boring yet amazingly nourishing meal.

▶ This rustic, comforting breakfast that's high in calcium and vitamin C can be fancified by topping with a smidgen of red pepper flakes and lemon zest before serving.

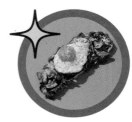

Kate's Mushroom & Greens Toast

✕

Serves: 2
Total: 15 min

▶ Heat 1 Tbsp **olive oil** in a large skillet on medium-high. Cook 10 oz **mixed mushrooms,** quartered if large, in 2 batches until golden brown, 4 to 6 minutes. Season with **salt** and **pepper** and transfer to a plate. Lower heat to medium. Add 4 cups **greens** and a drizzle of **olive oil,** season with salt and pepper, and cook, tossing until beginning to wilt, 1 to 3 minutes; remove from heat. Heat 2 tsp **olive oil** in a skillet on medium, and cook 2 large **eggs,** about 3 minutes for sunny-side up and over easy. Place 2 thick slices of **bread,** toasted, on plates, drizzle with oil, top with greens and grated **Parmesan,** then top with mushrooms and egg.

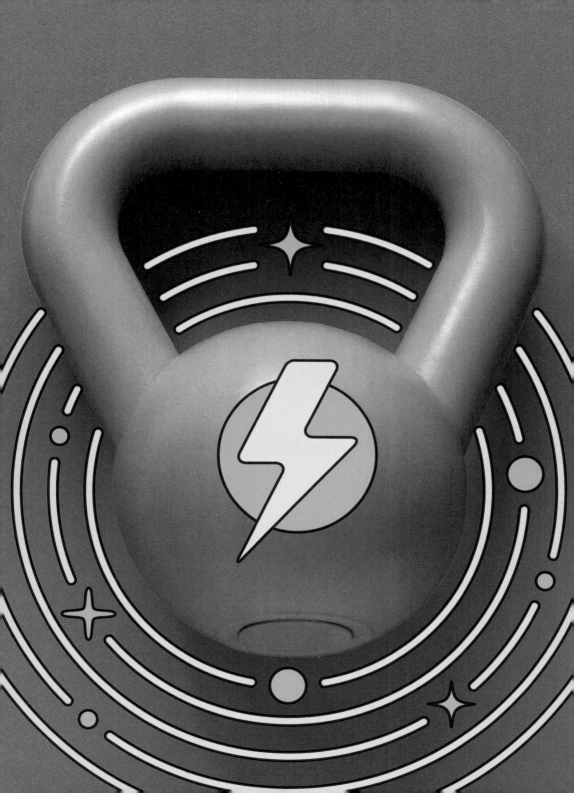

5

Sweat Changes Everything

A morning workout may be the most powerful thing you do all day.

Whether you're a first-timer, back at it after a break, or a committed gym-goer, I'm psyched that you want to make movement a nonnegotiable. *Really*. Seeing people click with fitness is hugely happy for me. Think of these tips as the wind behind you, pushing you forward toward your goals...and some amazing endorphins.

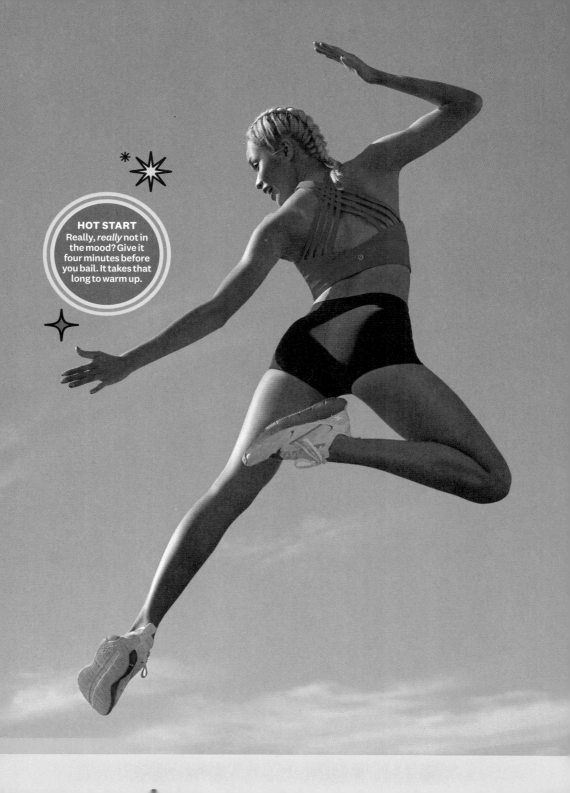

HOT START
Really, *really* not in the mood? Give it four minutes before you bail. It takes that long to warm up.

You're Always Better for It

We have a motto at *Women's Health*, which I firmly subscribe to: Sweat changes everything.
The magic of movement is real! Activity transforms your body chemistry, elevating your mood, increasing neuron activity, boosting your immune system, and reducing anxiety.

That's why most of my mornings include some form of fitness. It might mean a run in the park near my apartment or a weight-training routine at my neighborhood YMCA or even just some jumping jacks and core work right in my living room. Whether it's a little or a lot of sweat, moving my body makes me feel like a superhero.

I choose to exercise first thing because I want *alllll* of those positive benefits coursing through me for the rest of the day. If I've worked out, I am a better mom, partner, manager, colleague, friend, daughter...the list never ends.

But I also know that if I don't break a sweat first thing, it's just not going to happen. Yes, the obstacles of real life will pop up and get in the way. But the real reason I'm Team Mornings or nada? My motivation fizzles as the hours go by.

Having said all that, I understand that not everyone feels the morning sweat sesh. Totally fine! If you love a lunchtime or an evening (or a no thank you, not today!) workout, then don't force it in the a.m. Truly: Owning your morning is 100 percent about making the first few hours of the day the most powerful they can possibly be for *you*.

But! If you've tinkered with the idea of becoming a morning exerciser or wanted to sample the endorphin high that follows a sunrise sweat, I can assure you that it just gets better and better as your body becomes accustomed to the perks that movement unlocks.

The Science of Sweat

You know exercise is good for you. Ever wondered just how good? This is going to take a minute to unpack, because I want you to understand the positive effect that fitness has on your physical, mental, and emotional well-being.

IT MAKES YOU SMARTER

Workouts have numerous cognitive benefits, especially when it comes to memory and learning-related processes. One big reason: New neurons are generated by aerobic activity, as long as it's medium-intensity. More neurons means you can think faster on your feet and understand things more quickly. All of this has the bonus of making you less likely to develop brain diseases like Alzheimer's and dementia.

Plus, exercise triggers an increase in an important molecule called brain-derived neurotrophic factor (BDNF). Think of it as the maintenance crew making sure each part of your brain, from your hippocampus to neurons, can perform at its peak. High BDNF levels are related to enhanced spatial and verbal memory and recognition capabilities and may also counteract the effects of chronic stress. FYI: This book was almost entirely written by leveraging those dazzling post-sweat neurons. On the craziest of workdays, when I'll need my brain cells the most? Those are the morning workouts I never, ever skip.

IT LEVELS YOU OUT

I don't need to tell you that these are challenging times we're all living through. Whether it's craziness at work or alarming headlines, there are many reasons we feel frazzled on a given day. BDNF can keep your stress—and its unhealthy by-products, such as elevated blood pressure—in check. Just 15 minutes of aerobic activity two or three times a week can reduce anxiety significantly, per *European Journal of Sports Science* study.

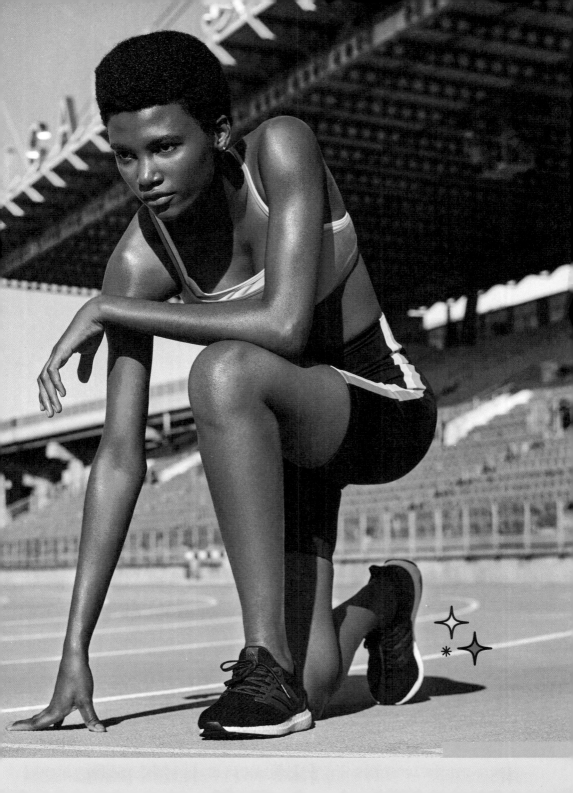

IT MAKES YOU MORE CONFIDENT

Sports psychologists have been studying the effect of aerobic activity on self-confidence for decades. And they keep coming to the same conclusion: Runners, cyclists, swimmers, and other athletes have high levels of it because of the sense of accomplishment they feel each time they cross the finish line—no matter where they fall in the pack.

You don't have to be a competitive athlete to reap the benefits, according to the researchers. (Phew!) Plus, with every rep you complete or step you take, blood and oxygen flood into your muscles, making them (literally) swell and look and feel extra sculpted. A-ha...no wonder I love a post-sweat selfie. *Feeling it!*

IT KEEPS YOU HEALTHY

Thousands of studies have revealed the various ways cardio and strength training improve our health: They lead to lower rates of obesity, heart disease, high blood pressure, type 2 diabetes, osteoporosis, stroke, and even certain types of cancer.

The heart-healthy benefits are pretty major too: A stronger heart pumps more blood with each beat, circulating oxygen more efficiently throughout your body; aerobic activity prevents inflammation; and lacing up your sneaks can increase the "good" cholesterol in your blood by up to 8 percent in just eight weeks, according to a study in the *Journal of Internal Medicine.*

IT BOOSTS YOUR IMMUNE SYSTEM

First, a moment of respect for your immune system, which fights all sorts of threats, from viruses to bacteria. Imagine you have an orchestra of instruments throughout your body— antibodies, white blood cells, bone marrow, the lymphatic system, and more—and exercise unites them in a symphony-level sync-up.

Scientists don't understand exactly how workouts mobilize this musical miracle, but they have theories. Exercise may help flush bacteria out of your lungs and airways, fending off colds and the flu, for example.

Physical activity causes a change in antibodies and white blood cells, which fight disease, circulating more rapidly after exercise. These speedsters may be able to detect illnesses earlier. Finally, the subtle spike in body temperature during and right after your workout may help your body ward off infection.

No Time? No Problem

This is my go-to 10-minute workout. It requires zero equipment, and you can count it as cardio *and* strength. Try it on a time-crunched morning.

Full disclosure: It is mega-challenging! You can take the intensity down a notch (or a lot of notches) by swapping in squats without the jumps, pushups from your knees, and, of course, rest and water breaks as you need them. You've got this.

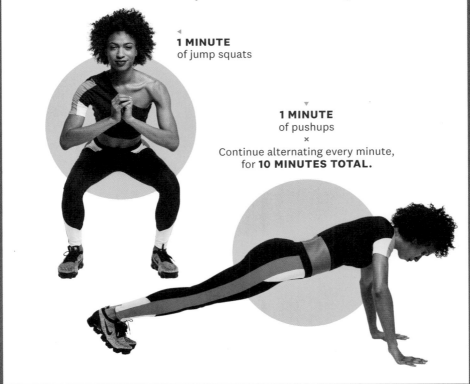

1 MINUTE
of jump squats

1 MINUTE
of pushups

×

Continue alternating every minute,
for **10 MINUTES TOTAL.**

Get Yourself a Goal

Everyone wakes up on the wrong (read: unmotivated) side of the bed sometimes. What to do? Set a performance goal. On those "I. Am. Not. Feeling. It." days, an extra boost is exactly what you need to get up and at 'em.

Make your goal something you think would be really cool to do—a handstand, nailing a dance routine, or, like me, a pullup!—then work backward from it to come up with a plan to get there. Keeping your eye on the prize instead of the clock can be the inspo you need to start a workout.

Once I put it out there that I wanted to achieve my first pullup—by telling, um, my Instagram followers—I committed to making it happen. There were many cold, dark mornings when it was tempting to snooze through my 5:17 a.m. alarm, but getting my first pullup inspired me to slip on my leggings and sweatshirt and sneakers for a trip to the gym. (I did eventually get my pullup—then promptly set a new goal to string together 10 in a row!)

Talking the talk helps me walk the walk, whether I want to push myself… or slow down. I shared that I wanted to run my fastest half-marathon in 2020. Which…nope. (Neither the 13.1 miles nor the PR.) But the sun and the moon continued to rise in the sky, and I don't regret putting my hopes and dreams out there, ready to soar.

So find your own form of accountability, whether it's sharing your goal with your friends and family, tweeting about it, hiring a coach or trainer to work with you, signing up for a virtual or IRL series of classes, or downloading a training plan. Or do a few things from that list. Share, plan, and get after it.

Any physical goal—as long as it's challenging, measurable, enjoyable, and achievable—will work, per studies. Nailing a complicated (or even easy, let's be honest) dance cardio routine? That would be neither enjoyable nor achievable for me—ha!—but you do you. The more specific you are about what you'll do to get there, the better it all works.

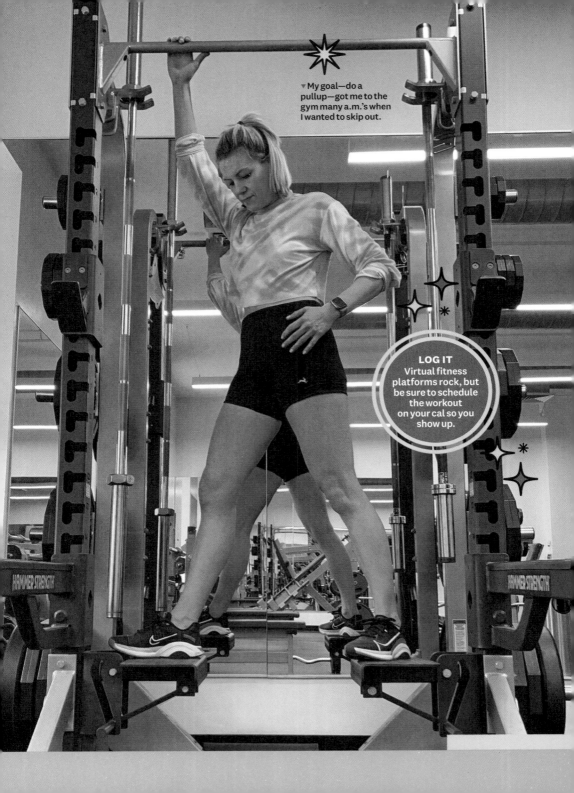

▼ My goal—do a pullup—got me to the gym many a.m.'s when I wanted to skip out.

LOG IT
Virtual fitness platforms rock, but be sure to schedule the workout on your cal so you show up.

Seal the Good Vibes

Take a minute to do a quick visualization. It's a sunny, crisp morning. You're nearing the finish line of a race, and as your leg muscles contract with each step, your lungs fill with oxygen, and sweat drips down your face, you can see the finish line in the distance. Now imagine the moment of crossing it. Your arms are extended high, a big smile stretches across your face, and confident, happy, feel-good endorphins zing around you like cartoon lightning bolts. Whether you've personally completed a 5-K or a marathon, you know the scene.

One of the most awesome and extraordinary things I've learned is that you don't need a "special occasion" to experience that energy. A quick workout followed by a personal celebration is all it takes. That's why it has become a tradition for me to finish every workout with a moment of celebration. My "victory dance" can take many forms: a high five with the person next to me in a class, an arm flex in the weight room's mirror, or a jump into the air after a run.

There is power in acknowledging that you just did something awesome, according to scientists. Accomplishments activate the reward center in your brain, which is what gives you a sense of pride. The neurochemical dopamine is released, creating a surge of feel-good emotions. (See? Those superhero vibes are not just in your head!)

It really doesn't matter how long or how hard you pushed—any effort is a win. Scientists call it "psychological momentum," and the TL;DR is that each victory boosts your overall sense of self-confidence, competence, and capability. The more wins you string together, the higher your expectations, and the more intense the mental and physical effort you put toward that task the next time. Positive momentum is a key to goal achievement and success, per studies.

Think of it as a little thank-you to your body. *I did that. I made it happen. Thank you. I appreciate you.* I often snap a picture of various "heck, *yesss!*" fitness moments using my phone's timer.

Admittedly, I have gotten some raised eyebrows from strangers at the gym and in the park during this ritual. But my photo app brims with smiling pictures of my flushed face and, yep, my flexed biceps, and I love each one.

A grateful scroll through them reminds me of all the endorphins I've been lucky enough to enjoy and how good my body feels when I give it the opportunity to move. Sometimes I even post these pictures to my Instagram feed with the hashtag #OwnYourMorning, in the hopes that they motivate one of my IG followers to get up and move...and then celebrate their workout victories. (Feel free to do the same and tag me @lizplosser—I'd love to see your pics.)

There is absolutely no need to photograph this moment, by the way. But please take a few seconds to acknowledge your workout win.

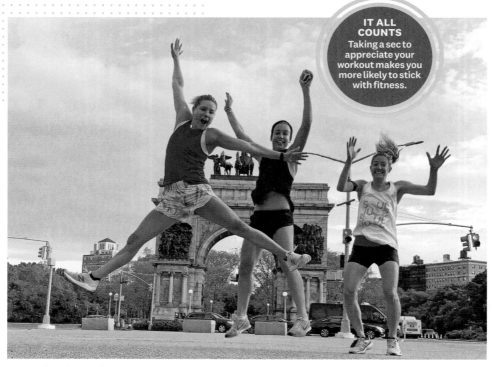

IT ALL COUNTS
Taking a sec to appreciate your workout makes you more likely to stick with fitness.

▶ My version of gratitude? Sharing a sweaty (jumping) selfie with my morning running buddies, Kelsy and Brooke.

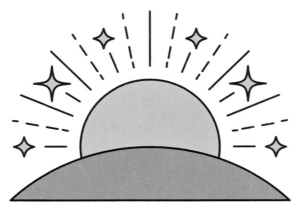

MORNING MAGIC

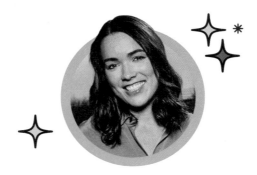

Abigail Cuffey,
executive editor, *Women's Health*

SOMETHING MAGICAL HAPPENED WHILE I WAS TRAINING FOR MY FIRST MARATHON...and it wasn't just my stronger legs and lungs. I found a brand-new (and incredibly effective, might I add) outlet for creative thinking and decision-making.

The time spent on my a.m. runs allowed me to really mull over a big idea or a major life change, and the repetitive activity served as a moving meditation. I started to notice that I made smarter, more measured decisions once I hashed it out—with myself—on a run. All the amazing endorphins aside, I'd end each run with a clear head and a path to a solution, one that really only presented itself in this sweaty situation. I fixed career obstacles, friend issues, marriage hiccups, and more while clipping along.

Ever since, I mentally press pause on a tricky problem or life question, waiting until my Saturday morning long run to play it over in my head. (Save it for the pavement!)

Even though my runs are shorter these days (I have a preschooler and a toddler, after all), I still break out this mind hack All. The. Time. And it's just as robust in smaller doses: Only 30 minutes of moderate activity was associated with better decision-making the rest of the day, found a study at the University of Western Australia. It might sound extreme, but I don't trust my initial gut feeling on anything until I give it this treatment: run, ruminate, react. It's yours for the trying—I can promise great decisions ahead!

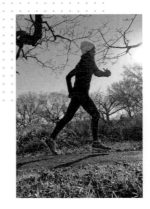

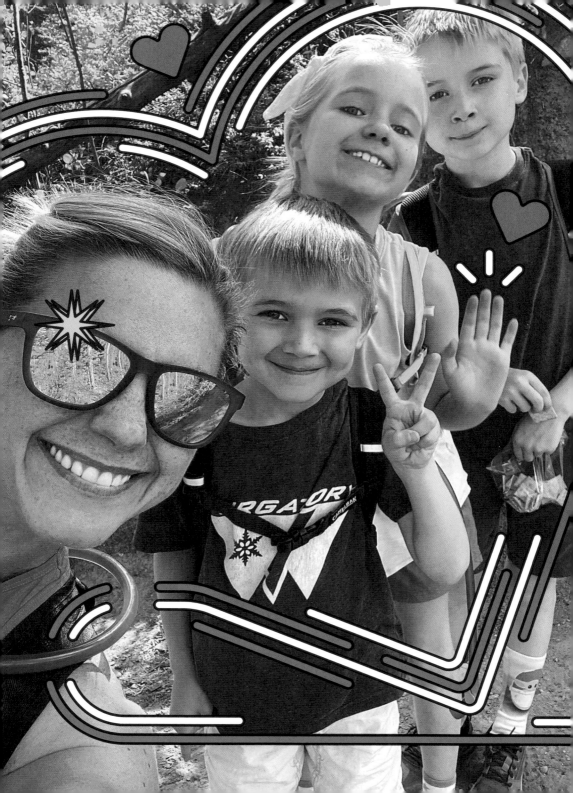

6

Even Stronger Bonds

**Make mini moments of connection
every single morning.**

Social bonds are essential to mental and emotional
health, and there are myriad effective, easy ways
to inject those important connector vibes into your life.
Ready for more of that good stuff? Same here.
Okay, quick, *right now*: Send a short text telling someone
you love that you are thinking about them. Feels
good, yeah? Now, let's explore how connecting with your
network is so important.

Go Ahead: Show the Love

My mom, who recently turned 70, is the brightest of bright lights in my life. She has taught me many lessons over the years, but the one I am most proud of embracing is her belief in expressing love—joyfully and often.

As a grown woman raising three young children with my husband, I am happy to report that I lead by my mom's example in the love and affection department. There is no shortage of hugs, pre-bed snuggles, and "I love you so much!" declarations in our household. One of my greatest joys as a mom is coming upon my kids holding hands or embracing (or petting/snuggling our dog, Willa) when they don't know anyone is watching.

To me, it's the ultimate parenting win, a confirmation that I've passed along everything my mom taught me. I get the same feeling when I see my colleagues virtually high-fiving each other on a job well done in our team Slack channel or when I see my friends commenting on each other's Instagram posts with a heart emoji. These quick acts of affection positively affect the recipient, the giver...and everyone who witnesses that transfer of energy.

Now, to interrupt this snapshot of unicorns-and-rainbows moments in my household with...mornings. The truth is that all the happy vibes seem to *whoosh* away once the hustle and bustle of getting out the front door on time kicks in. Our apartment becomes a tornado of "Where is my homework? Where is my shoe? There's no milk! We're late for the bus! No one brushed my hair!" Even on weekends, I bristle when I discover the kids on their devices playing video games before dawn. I turn into a major, um, Mom-ster. In those moments, our apartment becomes quite literally the opposite of Cuddle Land.

I set out on a mission to reframe my mornings as a celebratory capsule of time with my little Plossers. I felt extra motivated to do this because *family* (and the "full heart" part of my "clear eyes, full heart, can't lose" personal motto) is one of my core values. Yes, we're all trying to get out the door in our various ways, and yes, this time of day can be crazy. But it's also an opportunity to have a meal, catch up, play, and enjoy each other's company.

▶ Not pictured: the tornado-level hustle required to get all five of us out the door at sunrise for this epic Colorado hike.

It's worth noting that whatever your living situation, one immediate, universal impact of the pandemic that began in early 2020 was that most people reported feeling an intense sense of loneliness. An overwhelming sense of quiet crept into our lives, which we used to fill with city noises, trains, dates, parties, dinners, and more. But that loneliness also had an upside, which was that it allowed us to recognize the value of social ties.

The beautiful, magical secret is that we don't have to physically be in the same room to create connection and good energy. Mindfulness expert and mental health advocate Jay Shetty, the author of *Think Like a Monk*, felt this acutely at the height of the pandemic, when he and his wife were unable to travel from the U.S. to visit his family in London. "I learned that I could make them feel love, feel joy, and feel my energy if I really wanted to, even if it had to be done through a screen," he says. "And I could write them a letter. I learned that I could still say the beautiful things I wanted to share."

Whether you live alone or with a roommate, or you have kids, pets, or plant babies, you can create mini moments of connection with people you love and care about every single morning—whether they're nearby or not.

How to Create Connection 24/7

Willa is the Bernese mountain dog puppy we adopted in December 2020. I didn't think my heart could get fuller (it did), or my home more chaotic (also yes). My mornings with her gave me a new POV on friends and family: exhausting, but joy-inducing beyond measure.

CHALLENGE
TOUCH BASE WITH SOMEONE FAR AWAY

▼

OPPORTUNITY

Sending a 🖤 text with "I'm thinking about you. Have a wonderful day!" is a tiny action with big impact. Keep it simple and short. Doing something kind for another person not only makes them feel good but also elevates your own mood. Another idea: multitask. "I call my sister for a quick check-in chat while I'm walking my dog every morning," says life coach Judy Goldberg. Win-win.

CHALLENGE
CREATE A SWEET MOMENT WITH YOUR PARTNER IN THE MIDST OF RUSH HOUR

▼

OPPORTUNITY

Understanding how your romantic partner wants to be shown affection is half the victory. Maybe bringing a piping-hot mug of coffee into the bedroom for them would melt their tired heart. (It certainly would make mine sing!) Or perhaps it's about writing them a quick one-sentence note and tucking it into their bag so they find it later. Something like this: "I appreciate you! XOXO." Bonus: Gratitude (a.k.a. thankfulness) has been scientifically shown to boost your own mood and even impact your immunity in some cases. You know what would make your partner feel tingly and loved. Do that.

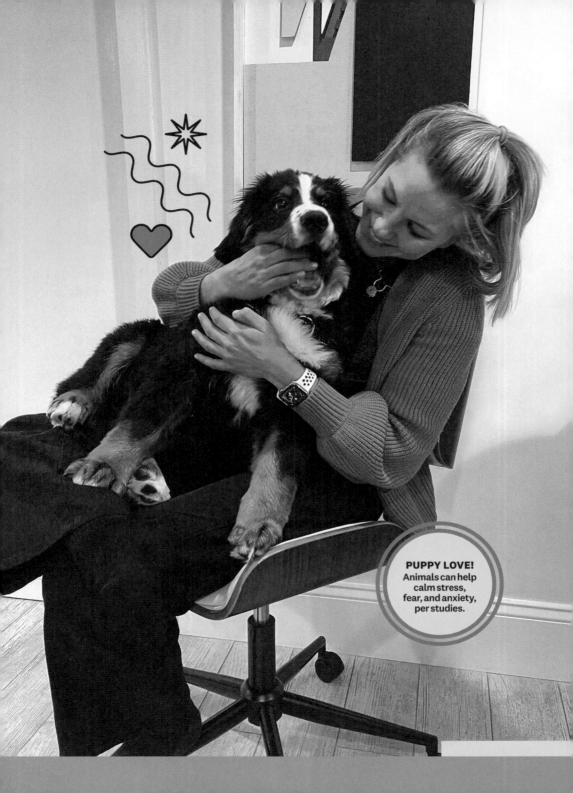

PUPPY LOVE!
Animals can help
calm stress,
fear, and anxiety,
per studies.

CHALLENGE
SHOW AFFECTION WHEN THERE'S NO TIME FOR SNUGGLES

▼

OPPORTUNITY
A quick kiss, a gentle squeeze, a big hug as your kiddo boards the school bus. I'm always on the hunt for these hidden moments...opportunities to sneak in a turbo version of a lazy Sunday morning cuddle sesh. Cool thing: Positive vibes are contagious (in a good way!), according to studies.

CHALLENGE
ASK FOR HELP

▼

OPPORTUNITY
When things are crazy, I ask the universe for a solid. "Please help me through this," I offer up to a nebulous higher power. (You don't have to identify as religious to do this.) Articulating a struggle helps me pivot in a positive direction. On a granular level, specify how those around you could help, like: "I'm feeling stir-crazy, any chance you have time for a morning walk?" to a friend. Or "I'm so stressed about a presentation; could you handle this staff meeting for me?" to a coworker.

✳

CHALLENGE
REIMAGINE A ROUGH PATCH AS A BONDING OPPORTUNITY

▼

OPPORTUNITY
Sometimes frustrating things just happen. You spill coffee down your shirt. You can't find your kid's show-and-tell object. You miss the bus. There's a traffic jam. On these days, I like to "clear the air" when I begin to interact with the outside world. For example, the NYC subway stops underground for 30 minutes, making me late to a morning meeting. I will enter the room and say (as calmly as possible), "I apologize for being late; I had some commuting drama." Acknowledging a tough moment without dragging everyone down into your basement of frazzle allows colleagues or household members to understand (and in almost every case, sympathize with!) why your energy may feel a little off... and it helps propel you all forward in a different direction. Being vulnerable and authentic (and, in the process, a lot more *relatable*), is highly underrated.

CHALLENGE
CONNECT ON A "DEEP" LEVEL WHEN TIME IS SHORT

▼

OPPORTUNITY

"The way we communicate and the words we use create energy," says Shetty, who is a big fan of upping your emotional vocabulary. "Most of us, when asked how we're doing, describe our life in four words: *okay, good, bad, fine.*" But a Harvard study found that using a limited number of words to communicate prevents us from diagnosing and expressing how we truly feel.

"We feel less understood by ourselves and by others, which makes us feel really disconnected from ourselves," explains Shetty. Challenge yourself to use more descriptive words—what psychologists call "labeling"—and encourage people you communicate with (colleagues, kids, friends, partners) to do the same. My kindergartner practices this life skill at the start of each school day with his teacher and classmates!

There is a colorfully comprehensive and helpful list of language developed by Harvard Medical School psychologist Susan David, PhD, author of *Emotional Agility.* You can find it by Googling "Harvard emotions list," and you'll be well on your way to developing deeper relationships.

Create Fun Communication Shortcuts

x

Clear, unambiguous interactions take a load off the brain, so Emily Anhalt, PsyD, cofounder of Coa, a mental fitness community, recommends establishing an emoji code with your friends or coworkers. A few ideas, below!

◄ **CACTUS**
It could signal a prickly subject that requires some extra tact and care.

◄ **BIG EYES**
Maybe on your work team it's a nod: "I see how hard you're working."

◄ **BOLT**
You could use it to convey excitement, as in, "love that idea."

◄ **LIGHTBULB**
When a topic needs brainstorming, from dinner takeout to a business decision.

◄ **CHART**
We're off to a strong start, but keep pushing: onward and upward!

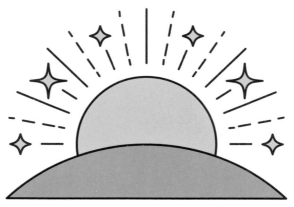

MORNING MAGIC

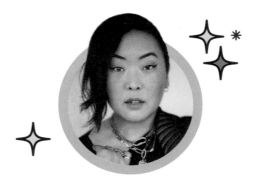

Aya Kanai, head of content and creator partnerships at Pinterest

IF I'M HONEST, there are times when "mom life" has been challenging because I am not able to click into "play mode" easily. I'm always planning our next event or meal and not as able to be in the moment as much as possible. My daughter, Rei, knows when I'm distracted by a work problem or my phone or just thoughts about life!

But mornings are when that play magic kicks in for me...and Rei and I are both here for it. It's always so fun to see Rei when she's waking up: I get to ask about her dreams and hear her first thoughts of the day.

Before working for a technology platform, I was a longtime fashion editor and stylist, so expressing creativity through what people wear is my expertise and my joy! Morning magic starts when I can talk with my daughter about what she will wear that day. I don't mean bows or frilly dresses; in fact, many of my daughter's clothes are gender neutral or hand-me-downs from a friend who has a son.

To me, creativity through fashion means talking about colors and textures and having fun with clothes and making outfits. Rei and I talk about tie-dye and pick from shirts with prints of pretzels, ghosts, and morning glories (her favorite flower), so it's a vocabulary lesson as well.

My mornings with Rei give me the opportunity to watch her develop preferences. (Now that she's a toddler, there are *a lot* of those, especially on days when we're late getting out the door.) These opinions are the building blocks of who we become. Expressing personal style has always given me pleasure... and it's amazing to see it forming and coming to life in a little person.

Creative expression isn't essential like food or water, but if you've ever seen a toddler spin around to show off an outfit, then you know it's pretty darn meaningful. That's the point: Style is not frivolous. Like music and art, style can make a good day a great one and also open the door to more creativity, satisfaction, enjoyment, confidence, and understanding. Which all means that a.m. playtime with Rei is the best part of my day.

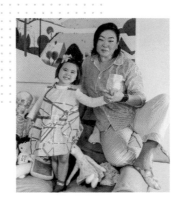

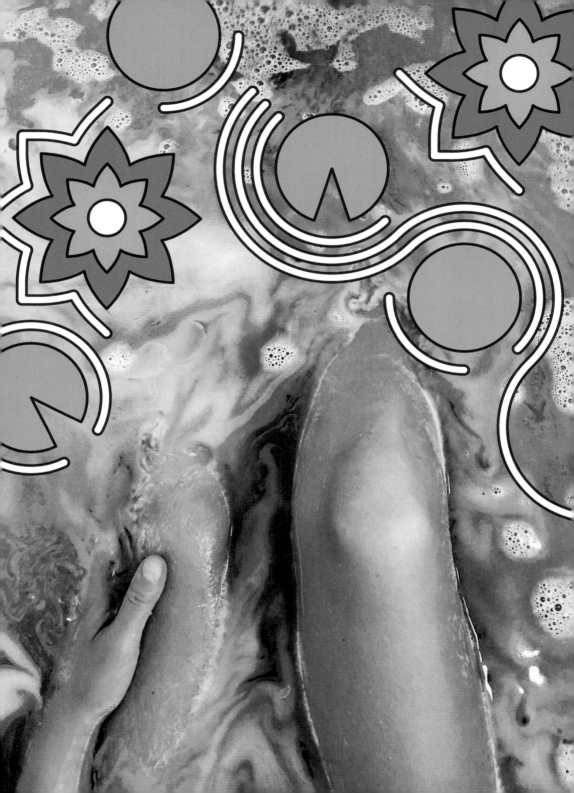

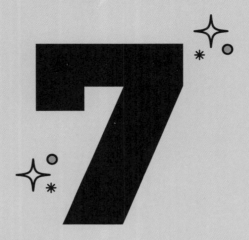

7

The Power of Meditation

Take a deep dive into the magic of mindfulness.
Imagine if there were a tool you could pick up to help you process emotions, allow you to be more present in your relationships, and strengthen you on your daily journey through life. What if it were free, and doable anywhere and at any time? You'd want to add it to your kit of life skills, full stop! I'm living proof that *anyone* can enjoy an impactful meditation practice.

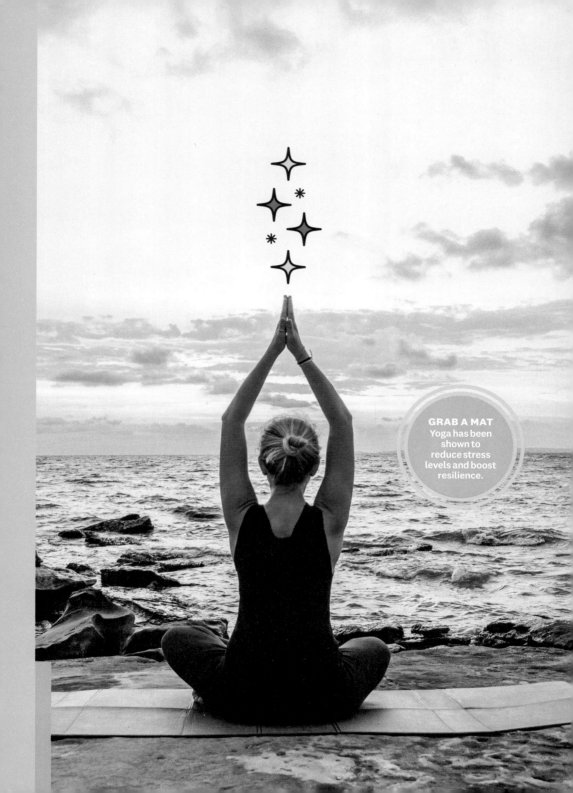

GRAB A MAT
Yoga has been shown to reduce stress levels and boost resilience.

Calling All Aspiring Meditators...

I attend a 60-minute-long yoga nidra session on Thursdays.
It's basically a guided-meditation-slash-zero-effort-required form of total-body relaxation. Given my complicated journey with meditation (more on that soon), it's pretty wild that I've carved out time for this regular practice.

A big reason why it works for me? Because it's led by my friend Georgia Rodman, a yoga and mindfulness instructor and the creator of the Spiritual Anarchy platform. She is all good vibes: Her soothing voice, her sage, colorful words, and her compassionate, uplifting energy swirl together to wrap you up in the equivalent of a warm embrace. Happy sigh.

As I actively work toward more mindful mornings, I'm lucky to have amazing mentors in my life, like Georgia, who show me day in and day out how powerful it is to bring reflection and curiosity into your personal world. Which is why I begin this chapter with Georgia's morning rituals, because #Goals.

She begins her day at 6 a.m. Rather than a standard alarm sound, chimes awaken her because "I don't need bleeping to start my day." She makes a cup of tea with a splash of milk, lights a candle, meditates for at least 20 minutes, writes a 10-item gratitude list, and then journals.

These rituals give her an anchor for the rest of the day. "I love the idea of showing up as a human being before I have to be a human *doing*," Georgia says. "Meditation sets a course of action. One positive action leads to the next." FYI, she also makes time to run through the woods for 20 minutes or to bang out a 30-minute HIIT session after this routine (movement can be a form of mindfulness too). Sweat changes everything!

It's Really, Really Good for You

For my entire almost two-decade career in the wellness space, I've heard about (and written about and edited stories about...) the power of meditation. There is indisputable, science-backed evidence that supports the health benefits of this modality. It has been shown to increase brain-wave activity—think: the daydream zone, when you're taking time off from a task—which makes you feel calmer. Meditation causes your adrenal glands to dial back production of the stress hormone cortisol. And it also increases blood flow to your brain, which may help lower anxiety levels while also boosting your memory.

This practice activates the area of your brain that controls complex thoughts and positive emotions while simultaneously lighting up the hubs in the brain related to feelings of compassion, empathy, and fear, giving you more control over your response to your emotions and helping you feel closer to others.

Studies have also found that meditation increases activity in your parasympathetic nervous system, which controls your rest-and-digest functions (the flip side of your fight-or-flight response). Reflexively, when you meditate, your lungs begin to draw deeper breaths. And your heart begins to beat more slowly, causing your blood vessels to relax. That's good news for heart health: In fact, regular meditation can drop your blood pressure by up to four points, lowering your risk for heart disease.

So yes, it's clearly very good for you. And yet! I will confess something regarding my personal feelings on meditation: I've had a little bit of a love-hate relationship with it. *Love* because I am *here* for anything that will help me live a healthier, happier life. And

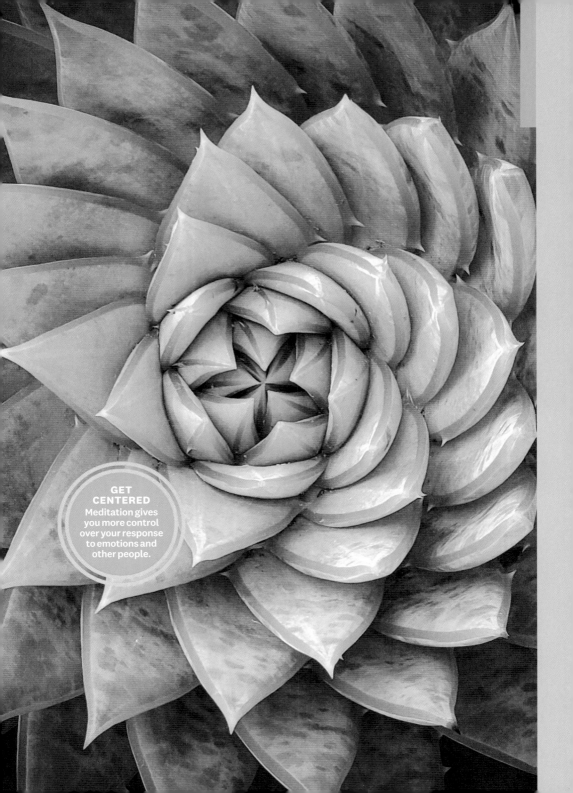

GET CENTERED
Meditation gives you more control over your response to emotions and other people.

hate because, well, I've never considered myself that "great" at it. A scroll through my App Store purchases over the years is illuminating. About every six months, I've downloaded an app with every intention that this is it, *this* is when I'll finally make meditation a regular part of my life. I log on once or twice. And then, poof, my resolve vanishes.

Thinking IRL meditation might finally stick for me, I even encouraged a former boss of mine (hi, Joyce!) to allow me to start a Meditation Club at a health-focused media brand I worked at years ago. I marched right into the reserved conference room and sat front and center for the first week, encouraging coworkers to leave their desks and join me along the way. But soon enough, I found myself dismissing the daily 11 a.m. calendar reminders and skipping another Meditation Club meeting because of my long to-do list.

I suspect this story resonates with others because I wasn't the only person who regularly bailed on the daily midmorning meditation. Within weeks, our 25-person-strong crew whittled itself down to two—two!—employees who conducted their own intimate meditation session together.

How much were we missing out on? A lot. But scoring the benefits of meditation is easier than I imagined, and it most certainly does not require a Herculean effort.

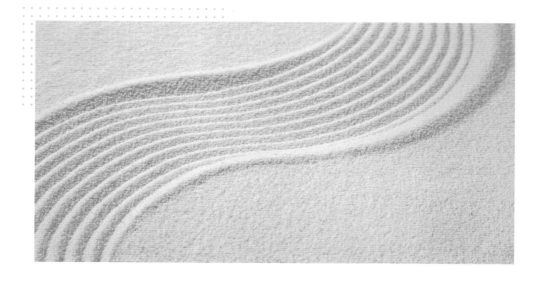

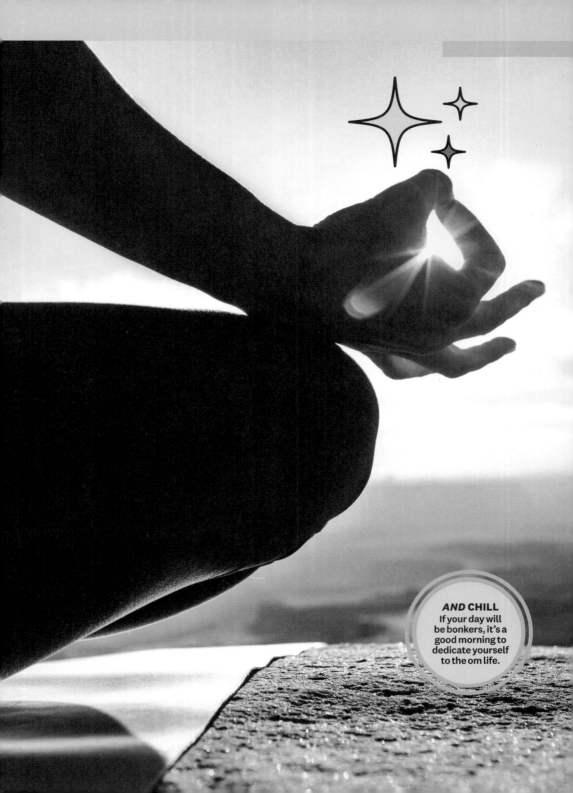

AND CHILL
If your day will be bonkers, it's a good morning to dedicate yourself to the om life.

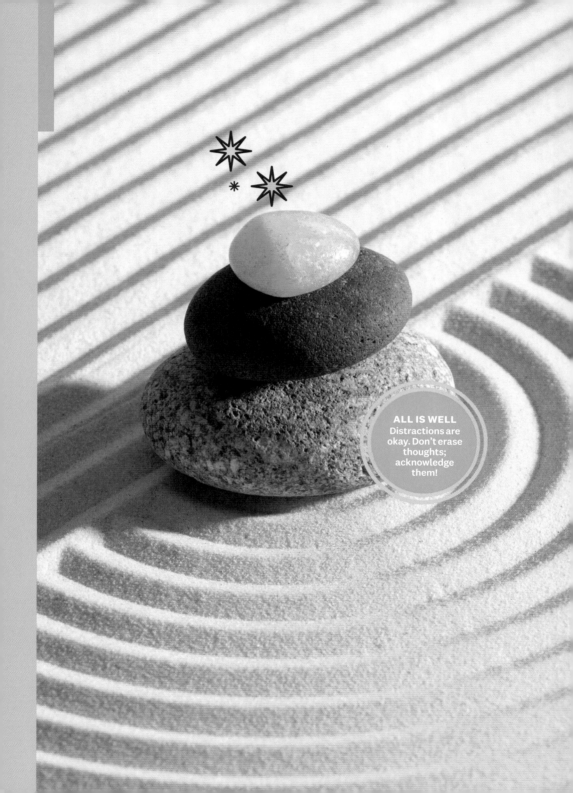

ALL IS WELL
Distractions are okay. Don't erase thoughts; acknowledge them!

Yep, *You* Can Meditate

•••

Jay Shetty is a mindfulness expert and the author of the best-selling book *Think Like a Monk*. A trained monk—who is passionate about normalizing the conversation around mental health—Jay is charismatic, magnetic, and oh-so-wise. "There are thousands of years of study around understanding the mind, human behavior, why we do what we do, how we can make better decisions, and where pressure and stress come from and how to actually navigate them," says Shetty. Enter: meditation.

▸ **FOR SHETTY,** meditation is the act of prepping your mind and body to take on the challenges of the day rather than entering it with fatigue, lethargy, and a lack of clarity. "The example I often give relates to sports," he says. (Shetty's superpower is explaining things in ways that will resonate with his audience....I've never met an athletic metaphor I didn't "get.")

"You don't 'train' when you're in the midst of the competition or game itself. You train during practice. And every morning, we need a training ground. We need a training center," he says. "Whether your training is 20 minutes or 10 minutes, or if it's an hour and a half, the point is finding your own space to try, stumble, and try again."

Jay meditates for 90 to 120 minutes on weekdays beginning at 6:15 a.m. (Goals, amirite?) But he encouraged me to think about the practice in shades of gray rather than all or nothing. "It's not about whether you do two hours or not," he assured me. "It's got nothing to do with that. It's so much more about you feeling like you're starting your day with your shield and your armor on so you're better prepared to deal with the challenges that are coming."

The more we talked, the more I realized that—without even knowing it—I had developed my own uniquely Liz form of meditation over the years. And even better, I was *already* practicing it at least twice a day! My version? Music.

How Breathwork Works

×

DEEP BREATHING CAN CALM YOU DOWN INSTANTLY

▸ **Basically, yes.** By manipulating your inhalations and exhalations, you influence your autonomic nervous system, which controls everything from your blood pressure to your hormones—ultimately, whether you're tense or calm, says Mimi Guarneri, MD, medical director at Guarneri Integrative Health. Even 60 seconds of deep breathing signals to your body that you're safe to relax.

YOU HAVE TO DO IT ALL THE TIME FOR IT TO WORK

▸ **Nope.** Since breathwork impacts your body so quickly, you can put it to use in the moments you need it, Dr. Guarneri says. In comes a stressful text message? *Exhaaale.*

BREATHWORK IS SPIRITUAL

▸ **That's up to you.** The concept of connecting with your breathing comes from ancient teachings that are spiritual in nature. (One example: Anapana meditation, a traditional Buddhist practice, involves focusing on the breath to help reach a state of wisdom.) However, breathwork can be a totally secular practice where you focus only on your physiology.

For the past couple of years, I've curated playlists for my morning commute from my home in Brooklyn to my Manhattan office. Some days, I need the audio version of a big mug of coffee: fast-tempo, toe-tapping beats accompanied by head-bopping, lip-syncing lyrics. Try feeling anything other than "Let's go!" when you DJ your subway ride with girl bands.

But other days, I want to take my high-adrenaline vibes down a notch. Maybe I'm hyped up over...just, you know, life. Nothing like some lovesick duets or moody ballads to chill me out and put things in perspective. I close my eyes, breathe deeply, and let the tunes reset me. By the time I take out my Air-Pods, I'm ready to bring the energy I've created to the people, places, and things I'll encounter that day.

That might mean getting my head right for a stressful work thing. But it also could entail finding a sense of peace on up-and-down days, or even unlocking some cleansing tears.

If meditation is a safe space to experience clarity, peace, shifting energy... well, then listening to music is my meditation. Yours might be gardening. Or making a pot of tea. Or even washing dishes. Maybe you sit down and bank a solid 15-plus minutes of traditional meditation, which is awesome too. It all counts.

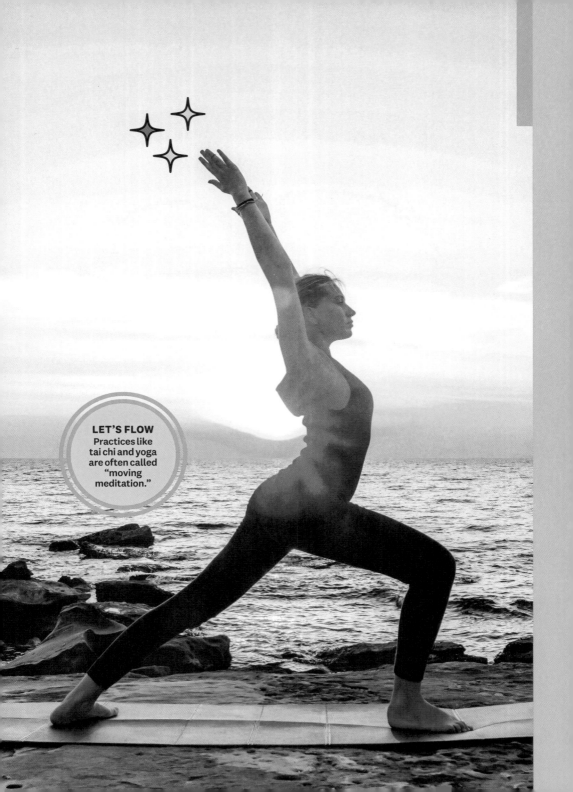

LET'S FLOW
Practices like tai chi and yoga are often called "moving meditation."

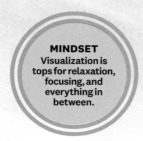
Jay Shetty's 5-4-3-2-1 Grounding Practice

•••

▸ **AS A MONK,** Shetty learned this technique, which is a favorite with psychologists and therapists alike. It is, essentially, a method of becoming present, aware, and attentive. When you are still with yourself, you actually notice what your body and mind want in that moment, and then you can go and find it.

Try this exercise and you might find that a few moments of mindfulness help you notice an ache in your leg that you haven't felt before, or you may realize that your lips are really dry and you want to drink some water, explains Shetty. The method not only allows you to listen to your body but sets you up to hear—really hear—those around you too. "If we're present with our body and mind, then we can communicate with our partners, our children, our colleagues, our friends."

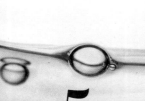

5

WHAT ARE FIVE THINGS YOU CAN SEE?

When you walk into a space, identify five things you can see. As I type this, I can see my laptop. I can see the ceiling. I can see the floor, and I can see the succulent on my desk. I can see my glass of fizzy water. Go through each and every one individually and patiently, taking deep breaths as you go.

4

WHAT ARE FOUR THINGS YOU CAN TOUCH?

Really experience them. Touch your shirt, grasp your chair, feel your ice-cold glass, click your laptop's keys. You may even notice sensations—maybe that the laptop is cooler than the chair, your shirt softer than the chair's cushion.

3

WHAT ARE THREE THINGS YOU CAN HEAR?

Take a moment to be really silent and try to become aware of what you can hear. It might be just white noise, or you may hear a bird distantly in the background. You may even hear other people in the next room. Listen.

2

WHAT ARE TWO THINGS YOU CAN SMELL?

Inhale and take a deep breath. What are those scents? Is it your cologne or perfume? Is it an essential oil? Is it fresh flowers from a loved one? Is something cooking in the oven? Take a moment to identify that smell.

1

WHAT IS ONE THING YOU CAN TASTE?

It might be coffee. It might be breakfast. It might be toothpaste. Identify it.

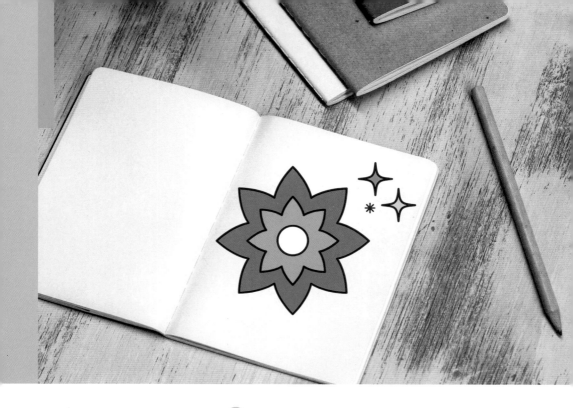

Anytime Inspo

Here are my two favorite journaling prompts, which always spark deep reflection and zinging clarity for me. Bonus: You can repeat them regularly because your thoughts and feelings are always evolving. Which is a beautiful thing!

1 GRATITUDE LIST Think back over the past week and write down things you are grateful for, big or small. There is no magic number, but 5 to 10 is where I typically land.

WHY? Gratitude is such a buzzword—and for good reason. Science shows that articulating gratitude makes us feel less anxious and boosts our mood. You can take things up a notch and create a list every morning.

2 SUPERPOWER Describe yourself as a video game character. Avatars tend to be archetypes—the hero, seeker, avenger, leader, etc. What do you wear? What do you wield? What is your name?

WHY? This prompt gives you an opportunity to reflect on your deeper values as illustrated by the avatar and its mission. It helps you define values that are important to you, whether you exhibit them already or aspire to develop them.

Mindfulness in the Palm of Your Hand

•••

These apps are tops for beginners.

HEADSPACE

▸ There are hundreds of guided meditations, mini meditations, sleep sounds, SOS meditations for emergencies, meditations for kids, and animations to help you better understand meditation.

CALM

▸ The app provides guided sessions ranging from 3 to 25 minutes, with topics from calming anxiety to gratitude to mindfulness at work—as well as sleep sounds, nature sounds, and breathing exercises—so you can really choose your focus.

INSIGHT TIMER

▸ You'll find experienced mindfulness teachers here, plus the freedom to pick and choose depending on how long you have to practice or what style you'd like (e.g., body scan, loving kindness, anxiety, stress reducing, etc.). You can also set a timer and sit without guidance.

AURA

▸ Fans of Aura like the daily meditations, life coaching, nature sounds, stories, and music, which are all personalized based on the mindset you select when you open the app. There's also an option to track your emotional state of mind and review patterns. And you can set reminders to breathe and take breaks for mindfulness throughout the day.

INSCAPE

▸ The main focus is reducing stress and anxiety and getting better Zs. Meditations, music, and breathing exercises are recommended based on your goals, the time of day, and your familiarity with meditating. It's a tailored experience, and even the names of the playlists feel hyperpersonalized (think Study Chill, Overcoming Your Fears, and more).

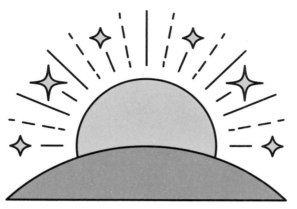

MORNING MAGIC

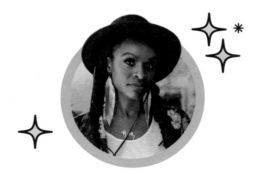

Latham Thomas, founder of Mama Glow,
a holistic lifestyle hub for women to
explore their creative edge through well-being

START EVERY DAY with a meditation practice called vocal toning. I play a note on a small instrument called a sruti box, then I hum with it a few times.

Instead of humming in a harmony or melody, it's just one singular tone that's aligned with the sound of my speaking voice. I like to think about it like an internal massage that I'm giving myself in the morning. It activates the vagus nerve, which originates in the brain and branches out in all different directions in the neck and torso, wrapping around every single organ in the body. Scientists often refer to this nerve as an "information superhighway" because it is involved in so many things in the body, such as controlling the muscles you use to swallow and speak, influencing your immune system, and even conveying sensory info from your skin.

This particular meditation practice allows for this feeling of what I like to call "attunements." It's like I'm tuning myself. The ritual, which I do for 10 to 15 minutes every morning, sets my day on a purposeful path. But it also serves as a reminder that I have a voice. And that I will use it!

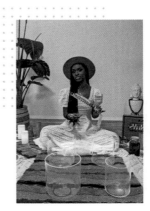

This is not a time for women to be silent. We're in a place where our voices are really needed. For me, my vocal toning meditation is a reminder of how I can be an advocate for someone, how I can advocate for myself and support my needs, but also how I can speak to injustice or things that are happening around me. It's a way of mindfully, purposefully setting my daily intention to use my power to do good in the world.

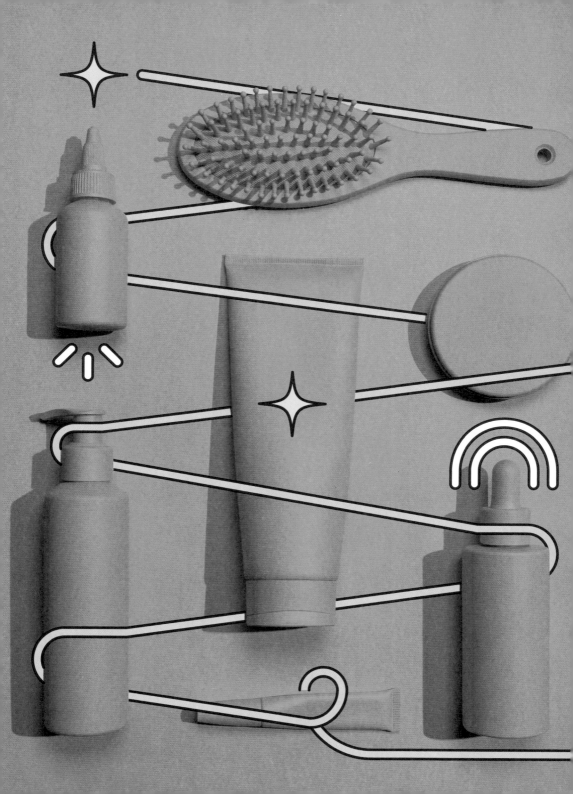

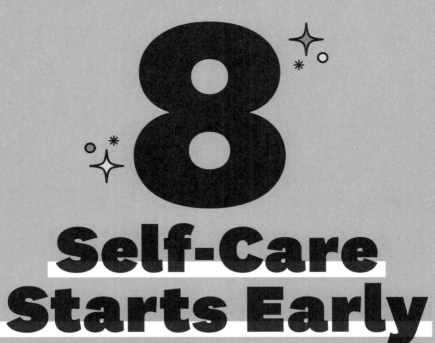

8
Self-Care Starts Early

**Skin and beauty rituals can make you
feel good inside *and* outside.**

My beauty routines lean more #MakeupFree than
#GlowUp, but I've learned that it's not really about how
many products I do or don't use. It's about building
micro-moments of personal maintenance into my morning:
taking the extra 30 seconds to mindfully massage a
serum onto my face, picking up the skin-care tool,
actually flossing, and so on. These little actions spark joy
and allow radiance to shine outwardly too.

Glow From Within

I learned a major lesson—*ahem,* understatement of a lifetime—while navigating the early days of the coronavirus pandemic in March 2020. My family effectively pressed the slow-motion button: We began working or attending school full-time from our apartment.

Without my usual morning structure to guide me, I found myself missing the hustle. Yes, even my commute on the crowded, almost always delayed NYC subway. Without having to rush to my kids' school bus stop at 8:04 a.m., I had more time and less focus.

And while I would never glorify how difficult that time was for everyone in the world, I also found strength in acknowledging the upsides, no matter how small. In that spirit: My skin-care routine flourished. I spent an extra couple of minutes massaging in eye cream. I layered on serums. I pulled out the jade roller that had been forgotten in a bathroom drawer. And wow, did my thirsty skin soak it all up. I swear my face looked brighter, glowier, and smoother every day. My husband, Matt, began joking that I was aging in reverse!

It's awesome to hear that you look extra amazing. But it's even more powerful to *feel* that way. My lockdown rituals of washing my face, brushing and flossing my teeth, and then applying moisturizer and sunscreen all helped me feel in control at a time when I had...none. And that's how a new form of self-care became a crucial part of my #OwnYourMorning routine, just like sweating and sipping coffee. On mornings I added a blow-dry and lip gloss? No question about it, I was next-level productive and felt more confident in Zoom meetings.

One reason I may have felt so good is because many beauty rituals involve physical touch. The sensation floods our bodies with feel-good oxytocin and activates the soothing centers of our brain.

This mainly happens in the hypothalamus, an area of the brain that's vital for hormone production, explains Jennifer Dragnet, PsyD, executive director of Newport Academy, a nationwide mental

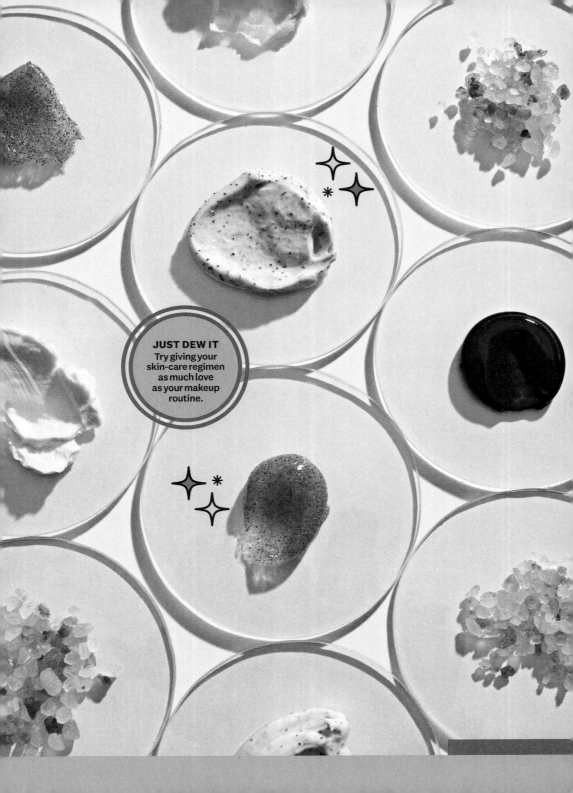

JUST DEW IT
Try giving your skin-care regimen as much love as your makeup routine.

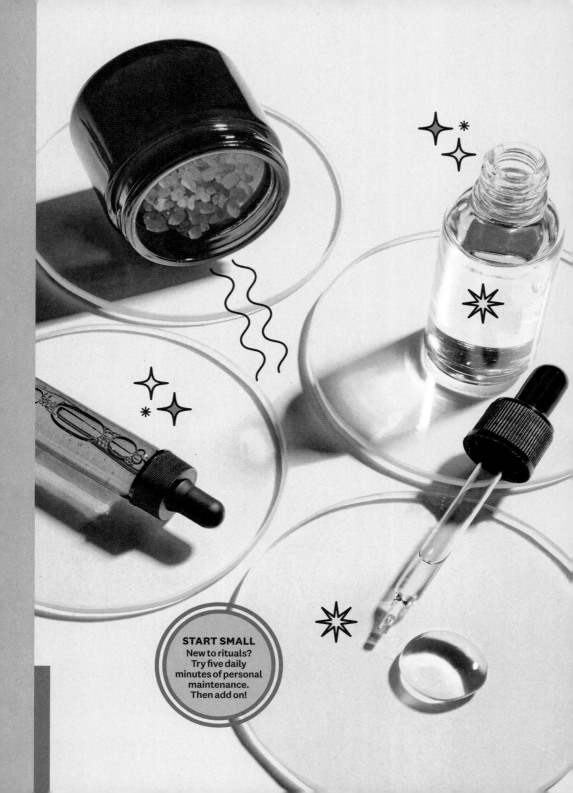

START SMALL
New to rituals?
Try five daily
minutes of personal
maintenance.
Then add on!

health treatment facility. It's similar to the happy high you get from petting a pup or finishing a yoga class. Here's how a morning beauty routine pays off—whatever is on your day's docket.

1 FEEL MORE IN CONTROL

Repetitive motions are particularly helpful in uncertainty because "we ultimately crave routine and structure in our lives," says Dragnet. "Even when it feels like the world is falling apart, taking a few moments for rituals reminds us we're in charge of our experience."

2 GET A POSITIVITY BOOST

You know those days you take time to do your hair and end up having more pep in your step? Yes, there really is something to it! "Taking a few moments to feel better about yourself can lead to greater self-esteem—crucial during challenging times when depression and anxiety increase," says Dragnet. Self-care rituals keep your spirits up. Committing to them shows you that you matter, which makes you feel better overall.

3 YOU'LL AMP UP CONFIDENCE

Not only will a dedicated routine help chillax you before a big day, but it can also lead to improved performance, per a *Journal of Organizational Behavior and Human Decision Processes* study. Laney Crowell, the founder of clean-beauty brand Saie, meditates while she masks and manifests everything she wants to happen in the day: "It sounds hokey but is really helpful for my mental health and productivity."

Make Your Routine More Like Self-Care

Your skin-care rituals, whatever that means for you RN, can and should be a delight, according to Alyssa "Lia" Mancao, LCSW. Her tips for blissed-out beauty:

× Single-Task It

"Engage in the activity with all senses," whether it's washing your face or applying makeup. Practice the 5-4-3-2-1 technique, which is described in detail on page 98.

× Linger Longer

If you normally take 30 seconds to apply a serum or face oil, set a timer and see if you can extend it a little bit. Slowing down—especially in the p.m.—helps your brain transition to wind-down mode.

× Clean Out Cabinets

Pare down and organize your products to reflect how you want to feel on the inside (clean and in control!). "If you're looking at a bunch of clutter, that's going to make you feel cluttered." Touché.

How ✦ Colors Can Affect Your Mood

Truth: Tints make you *feel* stuff: happier, calmer, playful, more confident. The hue of your clothing is a quick way to tap into the transformative power of the color spectrum. Leatrice Eiseman, a color specialist and the executive director of the Pantone Color Institute, shares the wardrobe inspiration you need to make moves... at work, in a workout, wherever!

WEAR RED TO FEEL STRONG AND CONFIDENT

▸ Tied to strength, red can boost your competitive spirit. There's a reason professional sports teams choose red jerseys. Try some crimson to nail a presentation...or your speed intervals.

PLAY WITH PURPLE

▸ The regal hue inspires experimentation. Add a bold pop of violet or a touch of lavender to your outfit before your next brainstorm sesh to get your neurons sparking.

CRUSH A FIRST IMPRESSIO N IN YELLOW

▸ The color elevates your mood, energy, and overall happiness. (It's my fave color! Can't resist a hopeful ray of sunshine, in any form.) Slip on a lemony tone if you're meeting new people and want to kick it off on the right foot. Lighter yellows tend to cause people to respond more positively to you.

FIND A SENSE OF ZEN IN GREEN

▸ Surrounding yourself with nature helps lower anxiety and decrease depression, and it's possible to experience some of these benefits by just looking at green shades. Channel this sensation with pieces that have hints of green close to those of blue (think: even more calming).

PERK UP WITH PINK

▸ If you're feeling playful, reach for rose or magenta. Pink is not only a romantic color—great for days you're feeling flirty—but it also gorgeously reflects off all skin types, giving you a healthy glow.

WEAR BLUE TO FEEL EXTRA CHILL

▸ Frazzled/stressed/tense? Deep breaths. Blue hues trigger special receptors in your eyes that send a "calm down" message, which lowers your blood pressure and heart rate.

BLACK FTW

▸ To get into boss mode, embrace Darth Vader–inspired vibes. People who wear black appear more intelligent, as well as more attractive, according to studies. The result: soaring self-esteem, which is tied to better health.

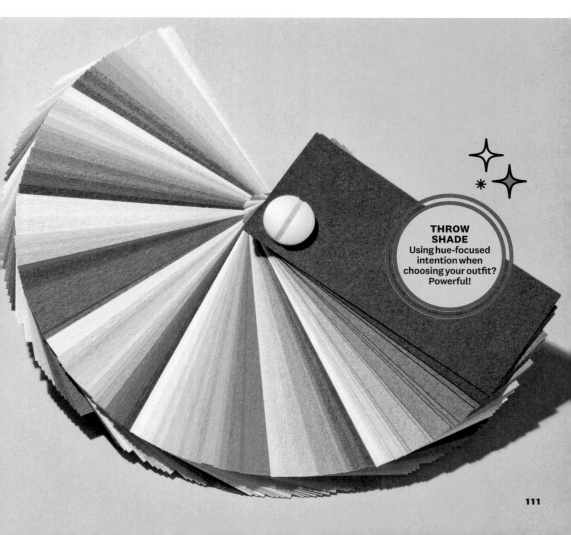

THROW SHADE Using hue-focused intention when choosing your outfit? Powerful!

Hair Hacks

I've had long hair since I was a toddler. Then a couple of years ago, I asked my stylist to chop it to shoulder length. Months later, I upped the ante to chin length. Although I sometimes miss the swish of my long ponytail, shorter hair has been a major morning game changer for me. I'm much more likely to blow-dry it after my post-sweat shower, and it's a cinch to style.

But the truth is that you can come up with a turbo routine no matter the length of your strands. Try these hair hacks from professional athletes with all different hair types.

FIND A GO-TO HAIRSTYLE UNIFORM

You don't want to fuss with a new 'do every day, so figure out one you can keep. In other words, set-it-and-forget-it hair. Soccer player Crystal Dunn of the U.S. Women's National Team wears cornrows in the summer because they require less upkeep. "They protect my hair from sun and sweat damage," she says. "I wear my hair in a variety of braided styles because it allows me to be creative and experiment."

REHAB WITH PANTRY STAPLES

As a triathlete, Gwen Jorgensen is very familiar with fighting the elements, like UV rays beaming down and drying out her strands. "For conditioner, once a week, I'll just use a simple coconut oil to rehydrate and smooth," she says. "I apply that before bed, sleep with it in, then rinse out in the shower after my morning run."

EMBRACE SECOND-OR THIRD-DAY HAIR

Skipping wash days is the key to a sporty updo, according to Kelley O'Hara, a soccer pro who plays defender. "I like my hair a little dirty because it stays better in a ponytail, and flyaways and baby hairs are kept down and back, out of my eyes," she says. Two days before a game, she shampoos and conditions; after practice the night before, she'll skip shampoo and only condition. This method leaves some sweat on strands for added texture.

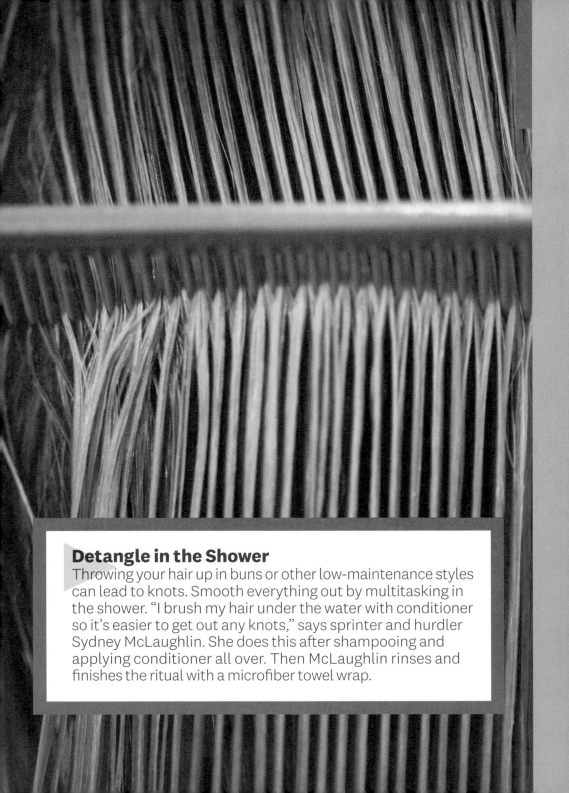

Detangle in the Shower

Throwing your hair up in buns or other low-maintenance styles can lead to knots. Smooth everything out by multitasking in the shower. "I brush my hair under the water with conditioner so it's easier to get out any knots," says sprinter and hurdler Sydney McLaughlin. She does this after shampooing and applying conditioner all over. Then McLaughlin rinses and finishes the ritual with a microfiber towel wrap.

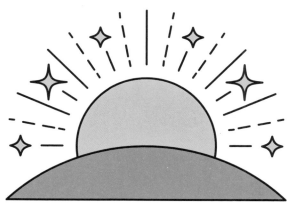

MORNING MAGIC

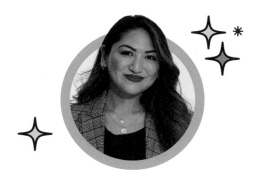

Kristina Rodulfo,
beauty director, *Women's Health*

NOTHING CAN GET BETWEEN ME and my morning facial skin-care routine. But when it comes to body care...I get lazy. That is, until I decided to change my habits by taking up a long-heralded practice: dry brushing.

"The main purpose is light exfoliation," says Hope Mitchell, MD, a dermatologist in Ohio. Layers of dead skin cells can block product (like lotion) absorption, so dry brushing helps you get "hydrated, silky, and glowing skin," she says.

Before my morning shower, I rub the firm, stiff bristles of the brush against my dry skin in light, circular movements. I start from my toes and stroke up my legs, arms, torso, and back (thank goodness for the handle). The motion is satisfying and wakes up my skin—almost as if there's an invigorating "buzz" all over.

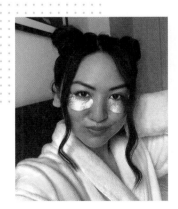

My skin looks and feels the smoothest it's ever been, but even more impressive? Several breakouts and leftover acne scars on my back completely cleared up (like, gone). Here's why: "Dry exfoliation followed by a shower will wash away dirt, oil, and those pesky skin cells that clog pores," Dr. Mitchell explains.

Considering it takes only a few minutes total, this pre-shower ritual has become my go-to way to kick off my day.

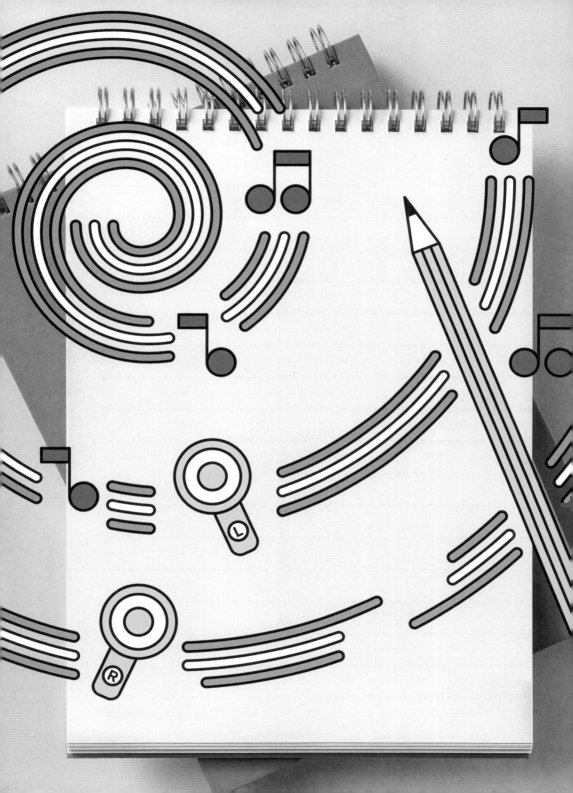

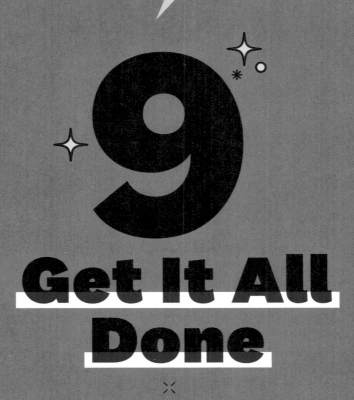

9

Get It All Done

Mornings are an ideal time to find your zone.
For me, that often involves work meetings. Once virtual calls became a normal part of the world, I learned pretty quickly that I could feel—and convey—energy over video platforms. I even began referring to it as *Zoomrgy* and *Slackrgy*. Eye contact and body language make a difference. I'd take it a step further and argue that you also absorb energy—good, bad, kind, anxious, invigorated—via devices. Here's how to make sure it's the positive, productive, twinkly-star kind.

Can an Inbox Be Joyful?

While sipping my first mug of coffee at the counter of my dark kitchen, I'm clicking through an average of four apps: Slack, the messaging tool my team uses to connect with one another; Google Analytics, the data platform where I check on *Women's Health* site traffic and top-performing stories; Outlook, my work email and calendar; and Instagram, my go-to spot to see what women are talking about in their captions and comments—it's one of my favorite places to find story ideas.

So yes, this is a decent amount of work before the day officially begins. Yep, it's a lotta technology at the crack of dawn. And yup, it works for me... though that doesn't mean it's right for everyone! Full disclosure: Occasionally, this routine will derail me and I'll end up scrapping my workout in order to crisis-manage something I discovered while scrolling. Luckily, that isn't the norm, and it's much more likely I'll happily simmer a request, idea, or

problem in the back of my mind while I sweat. And best-case scenario, it is resolved by the time my workout is over.

Sometimes I'll even set my alarm extra-extra early to practice a presentation, rehearse for a TV segment, or work on my monthly editor's letter. I know a lot of people are night owls who can own their evenings and the wee hours when there's a deadline hanging over them, but I'll always choose waking up a bit early the next morning over staying up really late.

And there is good news for those of us who aspire to maximize our early a.m.'s: How you handle the first few hours of your day can set you up for success the rest of the day, making you more proactive and better able to deal with what's thrown your way, according to research.

"A solid morning routine offers you control and peace of mind," says Mary Kelly, PhD, the CEO of Productive Leaders corporate advising. "That way, if something unexpected happens

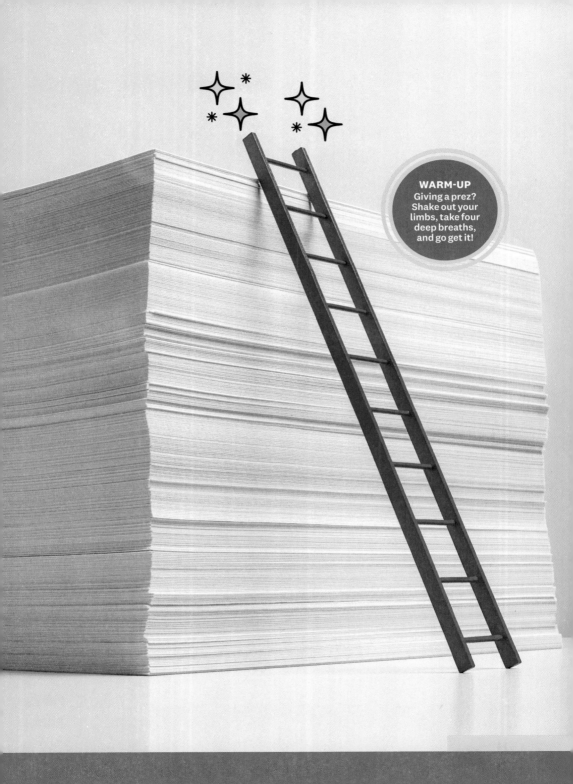

WARM-UP
Giving a prez?
Shake out your
limbs, take four
deep breaths,
and go get it!

later, you can flex with the situation. You've already taken the time to accomplish some important things on your to-do list."

Even better, science shows that we're extra primed to be productive, creative, and focused in the a.m., which makes it a great time to dig into a complicated project. However, that doesn't mean you need to start the grind before the sun's up. When researchers conducted brain scans of 900 people throughout the day, they found that participants were most alert in the morning, between 9 a.m. and 10 a.m. After that, markers of energy and efficiency decreased, and that was especially true after 11 a.m.

"You feel sharpest during the mid-morning hours, when you're rested and exposed to sunlight," says Daniel I. Kaufer, MD, an associate professor of neurology at the University of North Carolina School of Medicine. To put that brainpower to good use, schedule your most mentally demanding tasks on the early side and reserve your afternoon for email catch-up.

And whenever possible, try slotting in team meetings and important calls in the morning. Most of us are more easily distracted between noon and 4 p.m. than we are in the morning, psychologists at Pennsylvania State University have determined. So consider it the ultimate work hack: Stack whatever you want to be most focused, alert, and awesome for into your pre-lunch hours. Avoid the late-day brainstorm sessions and presentations when you can.

Speaking of things to sidestep, it's also a good idea to restrain yourself from doom-scrolling in the a.m. Reading alarming news stories can create an overwhelming sense of anxiety, according to multiple studies. "Our brains aren't meant to keep up with texts and headlines popping up on our phones constantly," says Mary McNaughton-Cassill, PhD, a professor of psychology at the University of Texas at San Antonio.

These pings tend to spike our stress levels, often sending us into fight-or-flight mode when, really, there's not much we can do about the situation. We don't fight, we don't fly away...we just sit there and stew. I don't know about you, but those are not the vibes I like to kick off my day with.

McNaughton-Cassill says you can avoid this unpleasant feeling by scheduling a "news hour" at a time when you tend to be more chill. That could be right after a great workout or during lunch; bad news is more disturbing when you're already anxious and tired, research shows. And consider this license *not* to check Twitter while eating your breakfast. Or before bed.

Open the Box

Before a virtual event at which I was a panelist, the organizers shipped me a very fancy, high-tech camera. They wanted panelists and moderators to have high-resolution videos in the livestream. That camera box? It sat there. I told myself: "I'm tech-savvy! I'll figure it out on the morning of the event, no problem."

What actually happened: In the hour before the panel began, I frantically tried all of the camera's settings, but nothing worked. And I didn't have enough time to ask for help or to troubleshoot.

So I swallowed the lump in my throat as my blurry Liz box appeared next to the crisp fancy-camera faces of my fellow panelists.

Ever since, "Open the box!" has become one of my favorite morning mantras. It's actually a lesson I first heard articulated by life coach Corey Anker. It's empowering to know what's ahead. So take a peek at the email. Open the PDF. See how long the form is. You'll save a lot of mental and emotional energy, and possibly even some midnight-hour anguish.

You don't have to put the camera together. Just take it out of the wrapping. Look at the cords. Flip through the instruction booklet. In other words, get started. This process not only sets you up to tackle and execute but also Just. Feels. Better. That's my approach to work and productivity in the morning. I hope you'll join me in the bubble wrap.

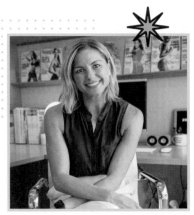

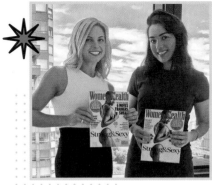

▶ Thankful for the energy the *WH* team brings to work every day. They make me want to soar.

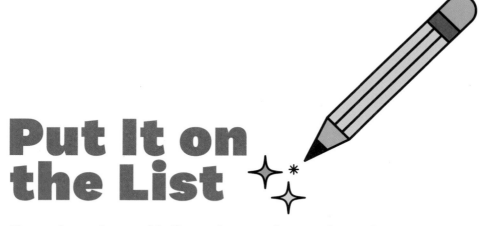

Put It on the List

I have always been a big list maker. I have notebooks, note apps, to-do list apps, Google docs, etc. brimming with various lists: what to pack for vacation, what to accomplish this weekend, what to finish at work today. As a gold-star lover, I find that feeling of drawing a line (or typing an X!) through/next to a task oh-so-satisfying.

And it's definitely not just in my head. Studies about goal-making show that an unfinished task causes interference—often unconsciously—with other tasks you're trying to complete. Translation: It's hanging out in your psyche, cluttering the mental and emotional space you could leverage in more productive ways. Also? It doesn't feel very good.

People with unfinished short-term goals performed poorly on unrelated reading and comprehension tasks, according to research in the *Journal of Personality and Social Psychology*. In other words, that presentation you need to craft could prevent you from giving 100 percent to other tasks. But there is a science-proven antidote: Making a plan to simply work *toward* that thing you're putting off helps your mind set it aside, freeing you to focus on other tasks. (I'm just talking about a list here—you don't actually have to complete the task.) When the study participants formulated lists of little to-dos, laddering up to their goals? The negative effects disappeared.

This is why I organize my to-dos into three buckets, a strategy I learned from my good friend Phoebe Jonas, an actor and life coach. Her method (described at right) helped me stop beating myself up about the length of my lists. It also gave me a road map to get my stuff done!

1

THE INDISPUTABLES

These are the nonnegotiables that must happen today. Try putting a time of day next to each one. For me, that means things like morning run at 6 a.m., making the kids' lunches at 7:15 a.m., school bus drop-off at 8:04 a.m., the 10:30 a.m. staff meeting, and so on.

2

THE MANUALS

I think of these as on-the-fly, where-and-if-you-can to-dos. Things like loading my credit cards into ApplePay on a new phone or updating the browser on my laptop with the IT desk. It would be great to get these done, but I'll squeeze them in when I can.

3

THE FLOATERS

These are tasks I'd like to complete in the next 30 to 60 days: a nonurgent email, a catch-up call with a college friend, picking a paint color for my daughter's bedroom. They feel amazing to finish but also shouldn't stress you out. Simply writing them down is enough for today.

EXTRA CREDIT

Add three open circles next to each item. Check them off as you begin (e.g., when you leave a voicemail), are mid-process (the meeting is scheduled), and, finally, completed (*yesss*).

Go With the Flow

●●●

You know that feeling when you're totally in the zone, everything's clicking, and the minutes and hours feel as if they're flying by? Scientists call it the flow state. And while you can't will yourself into this awesome mindset on demand, these hacks can re-create the brain activity that occurs when you're in the moment.

LISTEN UP
Playlists are my secret weapon to find my stride when I'm writing.

1
STOP MULTITASKING
In a flow state, your brain's prefrontal cortex (the decision-making spot) is less active, enabling you to focus on a specific goal. More distractions mean more prefrontal cortex buzz...and less chance of flow.

2
PICK A PROJECT YOU CAN SLAY
If you're working on something brand new to you, you're in learning mode, which activates the prefrontal cortex—the exact part of the brain that needs to chill out so you can find your rhythm.

3
FIND A PRIVATE SPOT
When your prefrontal cortex is less excited, it quiets self-analysis. Doing your thing solo offers the best shot of staying in that bubble where you don't wonder what others are thinking.

4
SHHH FOR A SEC
This helps you slip out of a beta brain state (adulting mode) into an alpha mode (daydreaming). Alpha brain waves help your mind move freely and can lead to a sense of effortless execution.

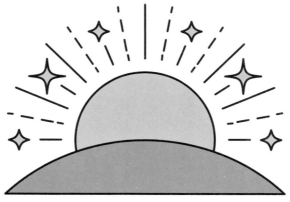

MORNING
MAGIC

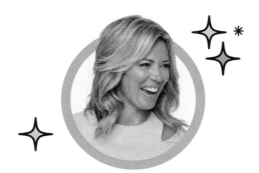

Brooke Baldwin, former CNN anchor,
Peabody Award winner, and author of *Huddle*

N MY LATE 30S, I had a lightning bolt moment: I can wake up my mind and body with purpose every morning to become a sharper journalist...and a better person.

When I was on live television for at least two hours every weekday, I never knew what was going to happen during that time. During any given segment, there were so many things keeping me on my toes. The teleprompter could go blank out of nowhere. News could break anywhere in the world. Throughout it all, I need to be gentle and deliberate in my delivery to a global audience.

That's why, early in the morning, I make it a point to move my body. Breaking a good sweat flips a switch inside of me. I lift weights, run outside, do indoor cycling, or take a virtual fitness class like Forward_Space (which is dance cardio) or The Class (which is high-intensity interval training plus a mindfulness workout in one).

Before I work out, I'm thinking about both the past (the news) and the future (my afternoon show, *CNN Newsroom With Brooke Baldwin*). That means mulling over different guests I want to book, angles for stories I want to cover, and how I want to frame a narrative that's shining a light on someone. Then, when I'm actually sweating, I'm trying to be present.

It's magic how each morning workout elevates my approach to work that day. Afterward, I'm so much more alert. And it lasts. I can still feel the focus and zing when I arrive at my office and begin to go over notes for my show. I'm just quicker...more attuned. While my hair and makeup are being done, endorphins are coursing through me, getting me ready to go live. By the time I sit in that chair on-set—and the lights go "bling!"—I'm 100 percent ready to turn it on.

If I don't work out? It feels as if I'm dragging myself around, kicking myself for not having done it. On those occasions, I've been known to jump around in my office doing burpees to conjure up some of those sweat vibes so that I can rock my show.

I love that by 8 a.m., I know I've already done the hardest physical thing I'll do all day. So throw anything my way. Bring it on, world.

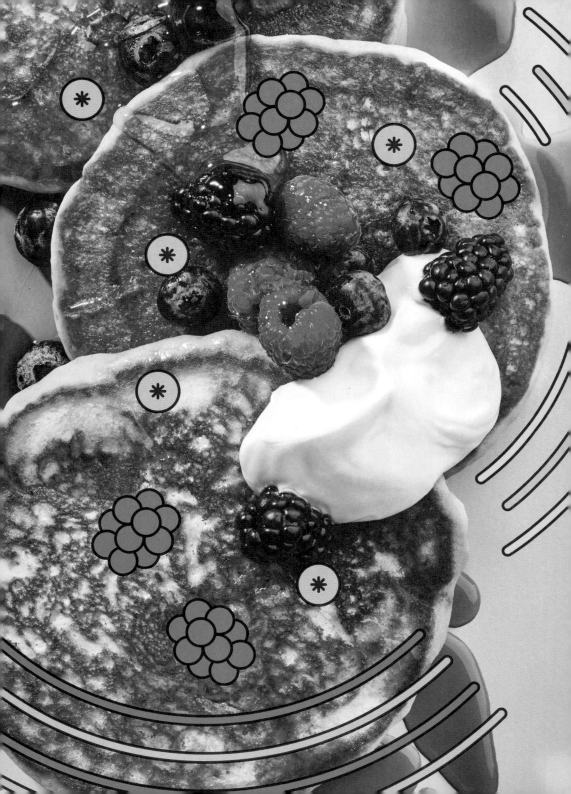

10
Win Your Weekend

Let's make the most of our "day off" mornings.
You have 48ish hours to recharge and reset so you can greet Monday energized and ready to rock. No winging it! Weekends require planning and thoughtfulness if you want to truly look forward to them. Think of these days as a mini vacation—which you'd never improv, right?—and you'll return to work happier, research suggests. Reclaim your time so you feel rejuvenated, over and over.

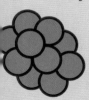

Recharge and Reset Yourself *

Just so you know: I'm not always up before sunrise. On weekends, I sleep as late as my kids and dog let me. I take advantage of the slower pace for indulgent moments: pancakes for breakfast, fancy products in my shower. I also bake in time to get a jump start on my workweek to squash the Sunday scaries, which 80 percent of workers report feeling, according to a LinkedIn survey.

I try to keep weekends sunny, at least figuratively speaking. I've found the best antidote to what scientists call "anticipatory anxiety"—that nebulous, heart-racing dark cloud hanging over the upcoming week—is a game plan. If you can follow this blueprint, you'll set yourself up for the best Monday ever. *Won*day, if you will. Because how you start your week is how you live your week!

1 DO THE BIGGIE BUMMER EARLY

Knock out your have-to-do-it-but-really-don't-want-to chores first thing Saturday morning. "Tackling your most dreaded tasks as soon as possible will give you a feeling of success early in the weekend and prevent anticipatory anxiety from stealing joy over those two days," says Katherine King, PsyD, an assistant professor of clinical psychology at William James College.

2 HAVE A BLAST

Listening to your favorite music while you fold laundry transforms a snoozefest chore into one that's semi-enjoyable. "Pair things you love with things you don't to reduce the burden," says Maria Sirois, PsyD, a psychologist who studies positivity. You'll soon feel less blah about your chores, or meet them with "less internal rejection," as Sirois puts it. Everything feels a lot bigger when it's stuck in my brain. Knowing which days/times I have big meetings,

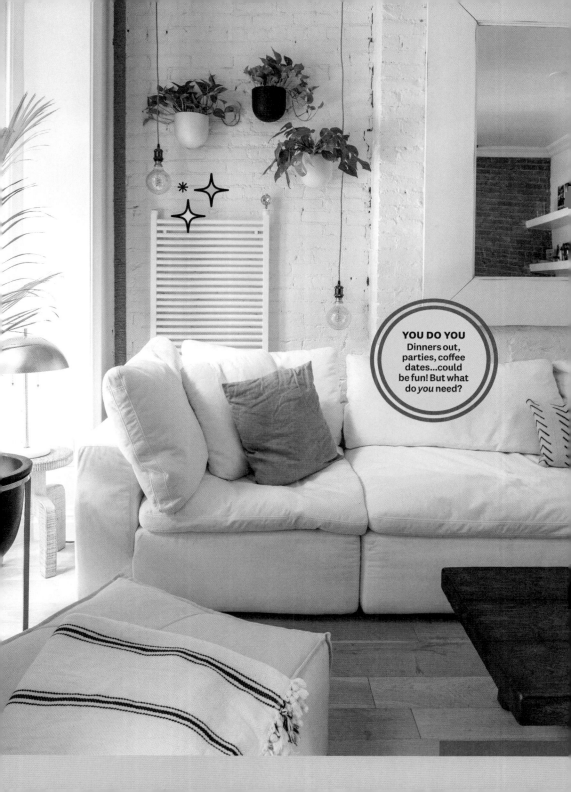

YOU DO YOU
Dinners out, parties, coffee dates...could be fun! But what do *you* need?

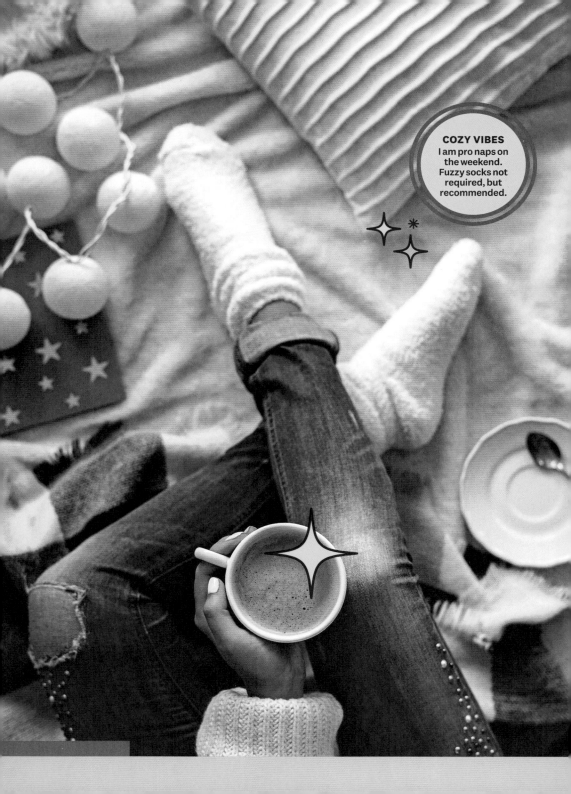

COZY VIBES
I am pro naps on the weekend. Fuzzy socks not required, but recommended.

deadlines, and more makes me feel in control. And the knowledge of when and what helps me stack my week accordingly: For example, if I'm doing a panel on Thursday, then I need to block out at an hour for prep the day before.

Writing and editing need interruption-free blocks of time, and if there's an upcoming due date during the week, I look out for myself and save time so I don't get overbooked with other meetings and obligations. TBH, proactive Sunday-evening calendar management is how this book got written!

3 BE A TIME-MANAGEMENT MVP
Figuring out how long tasks actually take is a skill to develop. So, for a month or two, track how long you spend on each to-do task. Once you realize the dishes don't take an hour and an oil change really might, you'll be better equipped to structure your days. To speed things up, stay present (no scrolling while you fold clothes!). "You're less likely to waste time when you're mindful," says Emiliana Simon-Thomas, PhD, a researcher at the University of California at Berkeley.

4 PLAN YOUR OUTFITS
I use the Notes app on my phone to track what I'll wear each day, all the way down to my kicks. I highlight factors that might affect outfit choices, like the weather forecast, TV appearances, or meetings that I want to be extra "on" for.

Sure, I may end up swapping something out during the week—usually the night before (see page 38)—but this gives me a running start on the week. It takes about 45 minutes and saves me at least 10 to 15 minutes of closet-and-laundry rummaging every weekday morning.

5 SCHEDULE YOUR WORKOUTS
Every Sunday, I text the girlfriends I run with to see which mornings they're free for some miles. Once I know which days we're meeting up, I build out the rest of my workouts. When will I lift weights at home? Do pullup drills at the gym? Is there a virtual class I want to try? I keep in mind which days it will rain, when my husband has to leave early for work, or whether I have big presentations. I reserve the right to change the plan based on how my body is feeling, but this fitness road map makes me so much more likely (and excited!) to set my daily 5:17 a.m. alarm.

6 PREP HEALTHY EATS
We're kind of obsessed with meal prep at *Women's Health*—so much so that we have a monthly column devoted to the topic. For some of our best weekend prepster tips, turn to "Ready, Set, Prep!" on page 134.

Ready, Set, Prep! ✶✦

Meal prepping allows you to cook on your schedule so you have home-made, healthy dishes on hand all week. But the thought of downing the same salmon, green beans, and quinoa combo four days in a row? Nope, nope, and nope. Enter: these smart strategies from the *Women's Health* food team.

ACE YOUR BASE

▸ Load up on pantry staples like grains, wraps, and breads, plus potatoes and hearty greens. Mixing up your meals will become a no-brainer.

PICK A PROTEIN

▸ Cook proteins in advance, and to prevent 'em from drying out, don't slice until you're ready to eat. And season simply so you're not stuck with spicy chicken for five days straight (been there, hated that).

CHOOSE A VEG

▸ In addition to your favorite raw salad options, choose hearty, versatile veggies like broccoli, peppers, sweet potatoes, squash, mushrooms, green beans, asparagus, and grape tomatoes. Cook them to extend their shelf life and you won't have to deal with a fridge full of food that has gone bad.

GO-TO GRAINS

▸ Leftovers last in the fridge for up to four days, and batches of brown rice, wheat berries, farro, and quinoa keep in the freezer for a month. To cool grains quickly, spread on a baking sheet. When you're ready to warm them, simply pop in the microwave for a minute or two.

PERFECT PASTAS

▸ Opt for noodles that taste good cold (looking at you, soba) so you don't have to deal with reheating spaghetti that's clumped together. For the same reason, embrace shorter pastas you'd find at a summer potluck, like fusilli or orecchiette, which tend to stay separated, unlike their longer siblings.

GREAT GREENS

▸ Water is enemy number one if you want to keep your produce crisp. When you're chopping and washing spinach or a head of romaine in advance, just make sure to pat everything dry. (Bonus for spin-drying first.) Buying prewashed? Check for moisture in the clamshell, and if needed, take out the greens and pat dry.

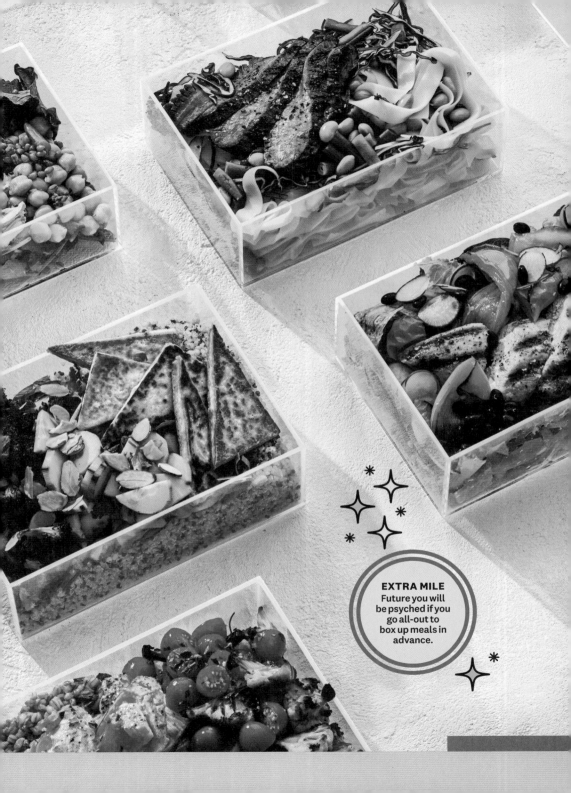

EXTRA MILE
Future you will
be psyched if you
go all-out to
box up meals in
advance.

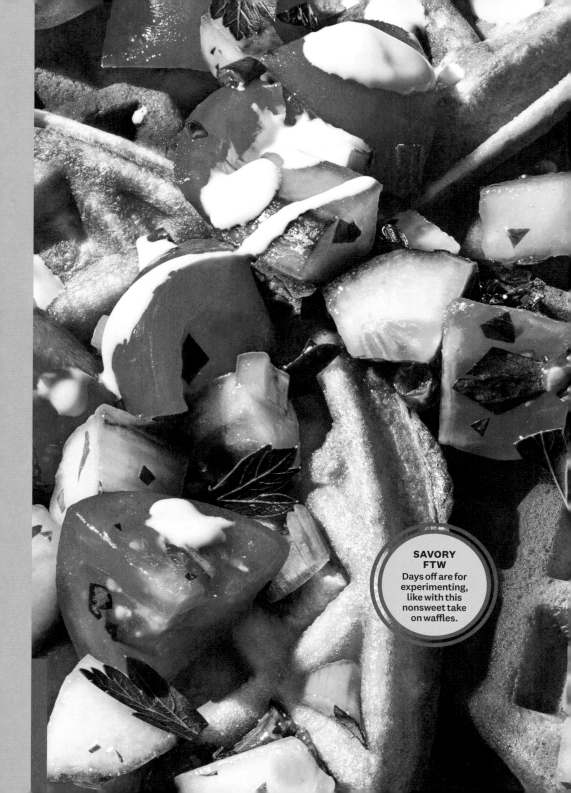

SAVORY FTW
Days off are for experimenting, like with this nonsweet take on waffles.

Weekend Waffles

×

These waffles are sorta like lunch—which makes them perfect for Sunday brunch!—and offer a hit of iron and fiber from the chickpea flour.

Serves: 4
Total: 30 min

▶ Heat oven to 200°F. Set a wire rack over a rimmed baking sheet and place in oven. Heat waffle iron per directions. In a large bowl, whisk together ¾ cup **chickpea flour,** ½ tsp **baking soda,** and ½ tsp **salt.** In a small bowl, whisk together ¾ cup **plain 2% Greek yogurt** and 6 large **eggs.** Stir wet ingredients into dry ingredients. Lightly coat waffle iron with nonstick cooking spray and, in batches, drop ¼ to ½ cup batter into each section of iron and cook until golden brown, 4 to 5 minutes. Transfer to oven and keep warm. Repeat with remaining batter. Serve topped with chopped **tomatoes, cucumbers,** and **scallions** tossed with **olive oil,** salt, **pepper,** and **parsley.** In a small bowl, combine yogurt and **lemon juice.** Drizzle yogurt sauce over waffles and serve.

Breakfast Burrito

×

Serves: 4
Total: 15 min

▶ Heat broiler. Arrange ½ lb **tomatillos,** husked, rinsed, and halved, and 1 **jalapeño,** halved and seeded, cut sides down, on a foil-lined baking sheet, along with ½ small **onion,** cut into wedges; broil until blistered, 10 to 12 minutes. Let vegetables cool, then transfer to a food processor. Add 2 Tbsp **lime juice,** ⅓ cup **cilantro,** and ¼ tsp **salt,** and pulse to combine. Beat 6 large **eggs** with 1 Tbsp **water** and ¼ tsp salt. Heat 1 tsp **olive oil** in a large nonstick skillet on medium. Add eggs and cook to desired doneness, 2 to 3 minutes for medium-soft eggs. Fold in ½ cup **Cheddar.** Spread 1 cup fat-free **refried beans** on 4 large **tortillas,** then divide eggs and remaining ½ cup cheese on top. Spoon 2 Tbsp salsa over each and roll burrito. If desired, crisp burrito in a nonstick skillet on medium. Serve with remaining salsa.

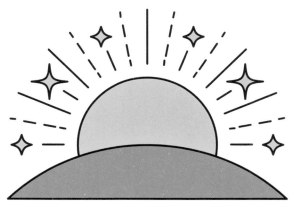

MORNING MAGIC

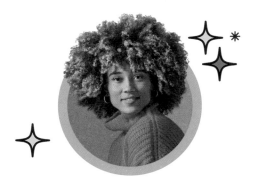

Ally Love, host for the NBA's Brooklyn Nets, Peloton instructor, and CEO of Love Squad—an organization and community that empowers women by providing affordable career support and inspiration

SUNDAY IS MY DAY. It's my favorite day of the week. I live in New York City, and I love the energy of being up early on a Sunday morning while the city is still asleep. It feels tranquil and inviting.

When I started as an instructor at Peloton (the at-home indoor cycling brand that streams live workouts every day of the week), they gave me, a rookie, the 11:30 spot on Sunday mornings. It wasn't exactly a coveted time, but I was thrilled! I knew I wanted the ride, which I named Sundays With Love, to be a celebration of life. I wanted to help give my riders an hour of total self-care—not just the physical aspects of a workout but also mental and spiritual self-care.

Each week, I focus on a different virtue and build the entire ride around that concept. Patience. Friendship. Hope. Faith. I explore different themes based on the time of year, holidays, or what's happening in the world. It takes extra work to plan and produce each ride because I'm going deeper and really trying to create a visceral response in my community. But it's worth it!

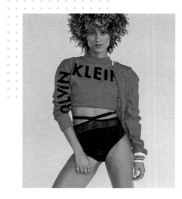

I've always believed that you can't be on E (a.k.a. empty) and give your best self in life. You can't fill up anyone else until you yourself are full. I know that in order to do my best work as the CEO of Love Squad, I have to nourish myself. And my Sundays fill me up. I never dread a Monday.

Index

Photo Credits

Kathryn Wirsing back cover (Liz in jumpsuit), **Becca Nelson** 15 (Maud Arnold headshot), **Natalie Ngo** 16 (Jeena Cho headshot), **Issey Kobori** 17 (Trinity Mouzon Wofford headshot), **Yumi Matsuo** 22 (Lauren Maillian headshot), **Kiana Toossi** 34 (Sofia Adler headshot), **Allie Holloway** 48 (Kristin Canning headshot), **Chelsea Kyle** 53 (coffee cups), **Mike Garten** 60 (Kate Merker headshot), **Danielle Daly** 61 (toast), **Martin Rusch** 64 (woman jumping), **Cathrine Wessel** 67 (woman about to run), **Allie Holloway** 69 (workout poses) and 74 (Abigail Cuffey headshot), **Renee Bevan** (Aya Kanai headshot), **Yumi Matsuo** 85 (Aya and her daughter), **Kathryn Wirsing** 102 (Latham Thomas headshot), **Jim Josephs** 114 (Kristina Rodulfo headshot), **Allie Holloway** 121 (Liz Plosser portrait), **Chelsea Kyle** 128 (pancakes) and 135 (container meals), **Sam Kaplan** 136 (waffles), **Danielle Daly** 137 (breakfast burrito), **Jay Sullivan** 138 (Ally Love headshot), **Caleb & Gladys/7 Artist Management** 139 (Ally Love full-body shot)

Getty Images: Alex Sava 4 (sunrise), **Di_Studio** 4 (bed), **Anton Eine** 4 (coffee), **Jenner Images** 4 (dumbbells), **The_Burtons** 4 (rocks), **Dannko** 4 (lemons), **PM Images** 4 (clock), **Arturo Rafael Enriquez/EyeEm** 8 (sunrise), **Samritk** 11 (alarm clock), **Blaine Harrington III** 12 (morning run), **LaylaBird** 14 (woman sleeping), **Patrick McMullan** 16 (Daphne Oz headshot), **Blaine Harrington III** 18 (cityscape), **Thomas Barwick** 21 (woman running), **Mohsen Ramezani-morad/EyeEm** 27 (fists), **Constantine Johnny** 29 (notepad), **Sutteerug** 36 (sheets), **Klaus Vedfelt** 38 (woman in sports jacket), **Adriano Pecchio** 39 (sink), **Somyot Techapuwapat/EyeEm** 40–41 (bed), **Xuanyu Han** 42 (night sky), **Newbird** 46 (feathers), **Eshma** 50 (coffee), **Claudia Totir** 54 (fruit bowl), **Kasia2003** 56 (toast), **JaneCocoa** 59 (coffee smoothie), **Tatomm** 62 (weight), **Aliaksandra Ivanova/EyeEm** 86 (bathtub), **Andrii Lutsyk/Ascent Xmedia** 88 (yoga on beach), **Melinda Podor** 91 (aloe), **Studio Doros** 92 (sand), **Jordan Siemens** 93 (meditating), **Wolfgang Filser/EyeEm** 94 (rocks on sand), **Andrii Lutsyk/Ascent Xmedia** 97 (yoga pose), **Biwa Studio** 98–99 (water), **Karl Tapales** 100 (notebook), **Lambada** 104 (beauty products), **Shana Novak** 107-108 (skin-care scrubs, two images), **MirageC** 111 (color wheel), **PeopleImages** 113 (hair), **Ko Hong-Wei/EyeEm** 116 (notebook), **PM Images** 119 (stack of paper), **Iordache Laurentiu/500px.** 123 (sticky notes), **PM Images** 124–125 (paper wave), **Cavan Images** 131 (living room), **Xsandra** 132 (coffee in bed), **Dimatlt633** 144 (pink clouds)

Courtesy Abigail Cuffey 75 (Abby running)
Courtesy Apple 83 (cactus emoji, eyes emoji, lightning bolt emoji, lightbulb emoji, chart emoji)
Courtesy CNN 126 (Brooke Baldwin headshot)
Courtesy Kristina Rodulfo 115 (eye mask)
Courtesy Liz Plosser 2 (Liz hiking), 4 (Liz and her kids, Liz jumping, Liz with dog, Liz and her husband), 6 (Liz on bench), 20 (two park images), 24 (Liz jumping), 30 (mood board), 33 (Liz jumping with sister), 71 (Liz in gym), 73 (Liz jumping with friends), 76 (Liz and her kids), 79 (Liz and family hiking), 81 (Liz and her dog), 121 (Liz and Abby)

HEARST
HOME

COVER AND BOOK DESIGN BY
Christine Demetres-Giordano

ILLUSTRATIONS BY
Mario Carpe

Library of Congress Cataloging-in-Publication
Data available on request

10 9 8 7 6 5 4 3 2 1

Published by Hearst Home, an imprint of
Hearst Books/Hearst Communications, Inc.

Hearst Communications, Inc.
300 W 57th Street
New York, NY 10019

For information about custom editions, special sales, premium, and
corporate purchases: hearst.com/magazines/hearst-books

PRINTED IN CHINA
ISBN 978-1-950785-70-4

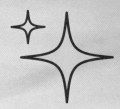